B LYMPHOCYTES

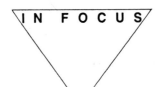

Titles published in the series:

*Antigen-presenting Cells

*Complement

Enzyme Kinetics

Gene Structure and Transcription

Genetic Engineering

*Immune Recognition

*B Lymphocytes

*Lymphokines

Membrane Structure and Function

Molecular Basis of Inherited Disease

Regulation of Enzyme Activity

*Published in association with the British Society for Immunology.

Series editors

David Rickwood

Department of Biology, University of Essex, Wivenhoe Park,
Colchester, Essex CO4 3SQ, UK

David Male

Institute of Psychiatry, De Crespigny Park, Denmark Hill,
London SE5 8AF, UK

B LYMPHOCYTES

G.G.B.Klaus

Division of Immunology, National Institute for Medical Research,
Mill Hill, London NW7 1AA, UK

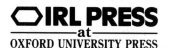
IRL PRESS
—at—
OXFORD UNIVERSITY PRESS

Oxford University Press
Walton Street, Oxford OX2 6DP

Oxford is a trade mark of Oxford University Press

Published in the United States
by Oxford University Press, New York

© Oxford University Press 1990

British Library Cataloguing in Publication Data
Klaus, G. G. B. (Gerry GB)
  B Lymphocytes.
  1. Animals. B-cells
  I. Title II. Series
  591.293
  ISBN 0-19-963191-3

Library of Congress Cataloging in Publication Data
  B Lymphocytes / G.G.B Klaus.
  1. B cells. I. Title. II. Series: In focus (Oxford, England)
  [DNLM: 1. B-Lymphocytes – immunology. 2. B-Lymphocytes –
  physiology. WH 200 K624b]
  QR185.8.B15K53 1990   599′.029 – dc20   90-4327
  ISBN 0-19-963191-3

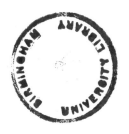

Typeset and printed by Information Press Ltd, Oxford, England.

Preface

The adaptive immune system evolved to provide a number of sophisticated defence mechanisms against pathogenic micro-organisms. The principal cells which mediate immune responses are T and B lymphocytes. B cells recognize antigens by means of specific cell surface antibody molecules. Some of their stimulated progeny produce circulating antibodies of the same specificity, whilst others develop into memory cells, which can respond more effectively to subsequent exposure to the antigen. The major functions of antibodies are to neutralize and ultimately eliminate native, soluble, or cell-associated foreign antigens; hence B cells are of particular importance in protection against bacterial infections. Recent years have produced rapid strides in our understanding of the biology and molecular genetics of antibody responses. Thus the molecular biology of antibody production is now well worked out. Considerable progress has also been made in unravelling the regulation of B cell activation by T cells and the cytokines they produce, and how micro-environmental factors determine whether B cells become antibody-producing cells or memory cells. This book therefore provides a timely review of our current knowledge of the cellular and molecular biology of B lymphocytes.

Gerry Klaus

Contents

Abbreviations

Ab	antibody
Ag	antigen
AFC	antibody-forming cell
APC	antigen-presenting (accessory) cell
BCDF	B cell differentiation factor
BCGF	B cell growth factor
Bm	B memory (or secondary) B cell
BSA	bovine serum albumin
BSF	B cell-stimulatory factor
CR	complement (C3) receptor
CD	cluster determinant (differentiation antigen)
DNP	2,4-dintrophenyl hapten
DTH	delayed-type hypersensitivity
EBV	Epstein–Barr virus
$F(ab')_2$	bivalent (pepsin) fragment of IgG Ab
FDC	follicular dendritic cell
$Fc\gamma R$	Fc receptor for complexed IgG
$Fc\epsilon R$	Fc receptor for IgE
HGG	human gamma globulin
$IFN\gamma$	gamma interferon
Ig	immunoglobulin
Id	idiotype
IL	(with number) interleukin (cytokine)
LFA	leukocyte function antigen
LPS	bacterial lipopolysaccharide
McAb	monoclonal antibody
MHC	major histocompatibility complex
OVA	ovalbumin
PMA	phorbol myristic acetate
PKC	protein kinase C
RaMIg	rabbit anti-mouse Ig
RGG	rabbit gamma globulin
sIg	surface (membrane) Ig
SRBC	sheep red blood cells

T_H	helper T cell
TCR	T cell (antigen) receptor
TD	T cell-dependent
TI	T cell-independent
TRF	T cell-replacing factor

1

Introduction

1. Adaptive immunity

Vertebrates deal with infectious agents by two broadly defined defence mechanisms: those that are innate, such as epithelial barriers, a variety of phagocytic cells, acute-phase proteins, and so forth, and those that are induced— adaptive immune responses. Adaptive responses have two cardinal features which distinguish them from innate defence mechanisms. Firstly, they are *specific* to the inducing agent. Secondly, the initial exposure to an infectious agent typically leads to the establishment of *immunological memory*. This results in the development of long-lasting, even life-long, immunity: re-exposure to the priming antigen leads to the production of a rapid, and often more effective, secondary (anamnestic) response.

The capacity to mount adaptive immune responses evolved into the sophisticated immune system now found in birds and mammals during the emergence of the vertebrates. The system can recognize an incredibly diverse array of foreign substances (antigens) and then generate effector mechanisms to neutralize, and ultimately eliminate, the antigen. A second integral feature of the immune system is its capacity to distinguish components of the body from foreign antigens (self – non-self discrimination).

1.1 Antigens

Antigens are substances capable of reacting with components of the immune system (such as antibodies). The term is often used interchangeably with the word *immunogen*, which more correctly refers to a substance capable of eliciting an immune response. Antigens comprise an extraordinary array of substances, including foreign cells, a wide variety of proteins (in native form or substituted with haptenic groups such as dinitrophenyl, DNP), polysaccharides, synthetic polypeptides, and so on. In short, antigens are molecules or associations of molecules capable of eliciting specific immune responses against one or more of their epitopes. A detailed discussion of epitopes (also known as antigenic determinants) is outside the scope of this volume. Suffice it to say that an antigen consists of an array of epitopes, which are chemical groupings which can be recognized by the antigen receptors on either T and/or B lymphocytes.

2. The lymphoid system

The cells which mediate adaptive immune responses are lymphocytes, which are distributed throughout the body, but which are particularly localized in the lymphoid organs. Primary lymphoid organs (such as the thymus) are concerned with the production of lymphocytes. Secondary lymphoid organs (the spleen, lymph nodes, and gut-associated lymphoid tissues) are where the cellular interactions resulting in immune responses largely take place. Lymphocytes are found also in many other tissues. Indeed an important characteristic of the lymphoid system is its highly dynamic and mobile nature, as the cells circulate from blood to lymph. This provides a widely distributed monitoring system to detect breaches in the integrity of the body associated with invasion by pathogenic micro-organisms.

The unique feature of lymphocytes is their capacity to recognize foreign antigens by means of cell surface receptors. Hence the essential features of any sort of adaptive immune response are

(1) the activation of clones of lymphocytes bearing receptors specific for epitopes on the antigen;
(2) their proliferation;
(3) concomitant differentiation into so-called 'effector cells' which actually mediate the response.

2.1 T and B lymphocytes

Lymphocytes in secondary lymphoid organs are highly differentiated cells, even before they encounter antigen. They are divided into functionally and phenotypically distinct subpopulations, which are specialized to fulfil particular roles in adaptive immunity. T cells need to pass through the thymus before they can mature into immunocompetent cells capable of recognizing antigen. B cells acquired their name because in birds they are produced in the *Bursa of Fabricius* (see Chapter 2).

Both T and B cells recognize antigens via their clonally distributed antigen receptors. The T cell antigen receptor (TCR) only recognizes antigens associated with cells of the host (such as components of viruses or intracellular bacteria). This is because the TCR binds peptide fragments of protein antigens which have become associated with cell surface glycoproteins (Class I or Class II molecules) encoded by the major histocompatibility complex (MHC). B lymphocytes, on the other hand, can recognize soluble, native antigens: they do this by virtue of antigen receptors on their surface, which are themselves antibodies (surface immunoglobulins, sIg).

2.2 Immune responses mediated by T and B cells

T cells and B cells undoubtedly evolved to deal with different forms of infectious agents. The division of the lymphoid system into these two major compartments of lymphocytes provides the cellular basis for *cell-mediated* and *humoral* immune responses. Cell-mediated (e.g. delayed type hypersensitivity, DTH) responses require the presence of immune cells and are essentially mediated by T cells. Humoral immune responses, on the other hand, are mediated by soluble antibodies secreted by the cellular progeny of appropriately stimulated B cells. One essential difference between these two arms of the immune system is that whilst antibodies can act at a distance from the cells that produced them, T cells need to directly engage the target cells of interest. It is thus likely that the B cell system evolved primarily to deal with soluble antigens. These can be cellular components of, or antigens released by, infectious agents. T cells, on the other hand, evolved to combat infections by intracellular micro-organisms, especially viruses.

B cells can respond directly to some antigens, in particular certain bacterial products. These so-called T cell-independent (TI) antigens are discussed in Chapter 3. However, the induction of antibody responses to most antigens, such as globular proteins, requires the interaction of antigen-specific B cells and a subpopulation of T cells called T-helper (T_H) cells. These T cell-dependent (TD) responses illustrate a striking feature of the immune system, namely that elicitation of the responses generally requires co-operative interactions between different types of cells (see Chapter 3).

2.3 Characteristics of B cells

B cells may thus be defined as those lymphocytes which carry clonally distributed sIg receptors for antigens which, when appropriately activated, proliferate and differentiate into end cells (antibody-forming cells, AFC, also called plasma cells) which secrete antibodies (see Chapter 3), or B memory cells, which can be re-activated by subsequent exposure to antigen to produce a second wave of AFC (see Chapter 4). The morphological features of an unstimulated B cell and of a plasma cell are illustrated in *Figure 1.1*.

In addition to expressing different forms of antigen receptors, B cells and T cells are further distinguished from one another on the basis of cell surface markers, which are generally membrane glycoproteins (see Chapter 2).

B cells in the secondary lymphoid organs are mostly found in dense aggregates called lymphoid follicles, whose functions are discussed in detail in Chapter 4. The B cells in lymph nodes and spleen are responsible for the production of various classes of antibodies after local or intravenous immunization, respectively. B cells in lymphoid tissues associated with the gut, respiratory tract, and various exocrine glands are predominantly committed to producing IgA antibodies (many of which appear in local secretions), and comprise part of the *mucosal immune system* (reviewed in 1). The T and B cells in these mucosal tissues display special migratory properties, since cells isolated from these sites home preferentially to mucosal tissues when re-injected into experimental animals.

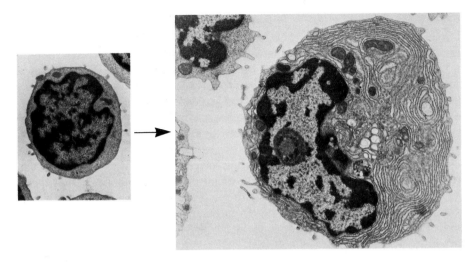

Figure 1.1.   Electron micrographs of an unstimulated B cell (left) showing the scanty cytoplasm with relatively few organelles, compared with a fully differentiated antibody-secreting plasma cell (right) with extensive lamellar endoplasmic reticulum. Courtesy of Professor A.Zicca and Professor C.Grossi.

3. Antibodies

The purpose of this book is to describe the biology of B cells. Before doing this, it is necessary to review briefly the characteristics of the recognition system used by B cells, both as cell surface receptors and as soluble effector molecules, namely antibodies. All immunoglobulins consist of one or more Y-shaped structures containing two heavy (H) and two light (L) chains, linked by disulphide bonds and non-covalent interactions. The N-terminal portion of the molecule contains the 2 antigen-binding sites (Fab regions), separated from the C-terminal portion (the Fc region) by a hinge, which gives the two arms considerable flexibility (reviewed in 2).

Antibody molecules are bifunctional. Firstly, they bind to individual epitopes on antigens with variable affinities. Then the bound antibodies can mediate effector functions, such as phagocytosis of the antigen or activation of the complement cascade. The effector mechanisms are brought into play as a result of the binding of the constant (C-terminal) domains comprising the Fc portion of the molecule to cellular receptors (Fc receptors, FcR), or complement components (such as C1q or C3). The antigen-binding sites of the molecule are formed by a combination of the N-terminal variable domains of the L and H-chains (V_L and V_H, respectively). The tertiary folding of the chains brings the hypervariable regions of the H and L chain together to form the contact residues of the antibody combining site.

There are 5 classes of immunoglobulins in mammals—IgM, IgG, IgA, IgD, and IgE—which have structurally different H chains (called μ, γ, α, δ, and ϵ, respectively). In both man and mouse there are 4 subclasses of IgG: in man these

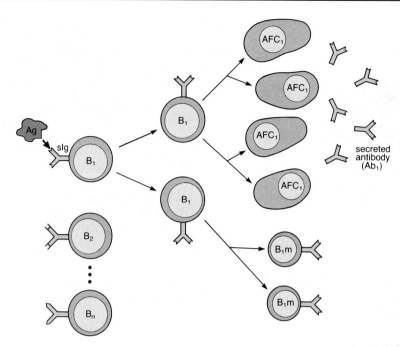

Figure 1.2.   Clonal selection. Gene rearrangements in pre-B cells generate the primary B cell repertoire with sIg receptors with specificities of $1 - n$. Immunization with antigen $(Ag)_1$ induces proliferation of B_1 cells, and their differentiation into AFC_1 (secreting Ab_1, top), and memory cells (B_1m) bearing sIg receptors of the same specificity as B_1 (bottom).

are IgG1, 2, 3, and 4, containing $\gamma1$, $\gamma2$, $\gamma3$, and $\gamma4$ H-chains, respectively, and in the mouse the subclasses are called IgG1, IgG2a, IgG2b, and IgG3. All isotypes share a common pool of L-chains, which can be either kappa or lambda. All classes of immunoglobulins can be produced during the course of antibody responses (with the apparent exception of IgD). Thus the circulating immunoglobulins (natural antibodies) found in the serum of healthy adults are principally the relics of previous encounters with a variety of environmental antigens. However, some may result from antigen-non-specific stimuli (such as bacterial endotoxins absorbed from the gut), which activate B cells to produce antibodies polyclonally (see Chapter 3). Furthermore, all classes of Ig can exist as cell surface receptors on B cells (see Chapter 2).

3.1 Antibody diversity

3.1.1 Clonal selection: one cell—one antibody

The total number of V-regions that can be made by all the B cells of an individual is called the *potential antibody repertoire*: it is estimated to consist of $c.$ 10^9 specificities. During B cell development (see Chapter 2) a series of gene rearrangements in the Ig loci result in the expression of sIg of a single specificity on a particular B cell (see below). A single B cell may carry more than one isotype of sIg on its surface (sIgM and sIgD being the commonest combination), but all of the sIg molecules on that cell carry the same V_H and V_L domains. The genetic processes leading to the generation of the antibody repertoire occur throughout life in the haematopoietic organs in mammals and lead to the development of a large number of clones of cells which comprise the *primary B cell repertoire*. Parenthetically, a similar sequence of events occurs in the thymus, to generate the T cell repertoire.

When an individual encounters a particular antigen this causes activation and proliferation of the clones of T and/or B cells bearing receptors of the appropriate specificities (*Figure 1.2*). This process is known as *clonal selection* and was first hypothetically formulated by Burnett in 1957 (3). The end result, in the case of an antibody response, is the production of circulating antibodies of the same specificities (i.e. bearing the same V-regions) as those of the sIg receptors of the B cells initially selected from the repertoire. The mechanisms involved in the antigen-driven phase of B cell differentiation are discussed in Chapter 3.

3.1.2 Mechanisms for generating diversity

Functional V-regions are the combinatorial products of 5 separate gene segments (reviewed in 4). The entire V-region is encoded by the combination of V and J (in the case of the L-chain), or V, D, and J segments (in the case of the H-chain). Estimates of the numbers of these gene segments suggest that if all V_H, D, and J combinations are possible, then combinatorial associations of these elements alone could generate $10^4 - 10^5$ V_H genes. A second source of diversity is the combinatorial association between V_H and V_L gene products. Thirdly, junctional mechanisms generate further diversity: these are due to recombinations occurring at varying nucleotide positions (and/or as a result of nucleotide additions) during the $V_H - D$ and $D - J_H$ joining processes. Similar junctional infidelity occurs during the generation of functional V_L in L chains.

The combined contributions of all these mechanisms are sufficient to generate the potential primary B cell repertoire of $10^8 - 10^9$ specificities. The shaping of the potential repertoire, and hence its relationship to the expressed repertoire, is discussed in Chapter 2. Finally, the primary V-region repertoire is known to be further modified through somatic mutations occurring in the V-region genes. This occurs largely after the cells have encountered antigen (Chapter 4).

4. Further reading

Roitt,I.M., Brostoff,J. and Male,D. (1989) *Immunology*. (2nd edn). Gower Medical Publishing, London.
Owen,M.J. and Lamb,J.R. (1988) *Immune Recognition*. IRL Press, Oxford.

5. References

1. Alley,C.D. and Mestecky,J. (1988) In *B Lymphocytes in Human Disease*. Bird,G. and Calvert,J.E. (ed.), Oxford Medical Publications, Oxford, p. 223.
2. Bird,P. (1988) In *B Lymphocyte in Human Disease*. Bird,G. and Calvert,J.E. (ed.), Oxford University Press, Oxford, p. 3.
3. Burnet,F.M. (1957) *The Clonal Selection Theory of Acquired Immunity*. Cambridge University Press, Cambridge.
4. Honjo,T. and Habu,S. (1985) *Ann. Rev. Biochem.*, **54**, 803.

2

The development of B cells

1. Introduction

The differentiation of B cells is conveniently considered in two distinct phases. The first phase, which will be discussed in this chapter, occurs in lymphopoietic organs. This encompasses the development of the immunocompetent primary B cell repertoire. The most important molecular processes that occur during this phase are the ordered sequence of gene rearrangements which result in the expression of clonally distributed sIg receptors on cells which then populate the periphery. In addition, the developing cells also express other cell surface glycoproteins characteristic of the lineage. This phase of differentiation is independent of exogenous antigen stimulation, it commences during fetal life, and in mammals it continues throughout the life of the individual.

The second phase of B cell differentiation is antigen driven: appropriate clones of cells selected by antigen from the primary repertoire proliferate and differentiate into AFC (see Chapter 3) and/or B memory (secondary) B cells (see Chapter 4).

2. B cell development in birds

One of the first indications for the existence of separate lineages of T and B cells came from experiments in chickens. Birds have a lymphoepithelial organ in their hind gut called the *Bursa of Fabricius*: surgical ablation of the bursa in early life causes a selective immunodeficiency in the adult birds in their capacity to produce antibodies, and leaves cell-mediated immune responses (such as DTH responses and the capacity to reject foreign tissue grafts) intact (1). The bursa is seeded by mesenchymal progenitor cells between the 8th and 14th day of embryonic life. Some of these progenitors differentiate into sIgM$^+$ B cells, which divide to form a large number of lymphoid follicles, and the B lymphocytes arising from these migrate to the periphery from day 16 of incubation. The bursa involutes when the bird is about 4–5 months old, having produced sufficient B cells for the lifetime of the animal. The genetic mechanisms whereby birds generate their repertoire of antibody specificities is different than in mammals. Chickens only have a limited number of V-region genes and generate diversity by gene conversions using pseudogenes (2).

3. B cell development in mammals

Mammals do not have a bursa: the gut-associated lymphoid tissues (e.g. tonsils, Peyer's patches, and the appendix) in mammals are secondary lymphoid organs, concerned with the generation of immune responses rather than with lymphopoiesis.

In fetal mice and humans the liver is the first site of B-lymphopoiesis: this commences from the 12th to the 14th day of gestation in the mouse, and around 8–9 weeks in the human fetus. In adult mammals B cells are produced in the bone marrow together with all the other blood elements.

3.1 Stages of differentiation during haemopoiesis

All the blood elements including B and T lymphocytes develop from a common, pluripotent haematopoietic stem cell. The nature of this cell is now fairly well established in the mouse (3). It is believed that lymphocytes develop from a common lymphoid progenitor cell, but there is little direct evidence for this. The first recognizable cell in the B cell lineage is the pro-pre-B cell, which has rearranged the V-region genes for the μ-chain (see below), but does not yet make the protein (*Figure 2.1*). This becomes a large, rapidly dividing cytoplasmic μ-positive ($c\mu^+$) pre-B cell (first detectable around day 12 of fetal life in the mouse). This cell stops dividing, becomes smaller, and over a period of some 24 h rearranges its L-chain V genes. As a consequence these cells express sIgM receptors and leave the marrow as immature B cells (reviewed in 4). Most of these cells go on to synthesize δ chains also (carrying the same V_H as the μ chain) and hence mature into fully immunocompetent peripheral B cells.

3.2 Control of B lymphopoiesis

It has been estimated that the bone marrow of an adult mouse contains about 3×10^7 pre-B cells. These produce approximately $2–5 \times 10^7$ primary B cells per day, which represents some 10–20% of the animal's total peripheral pool (5). The marrow therefore produces sufficient B cells to totally replace the peripheral pool every few days. Large numbers of B cells therefore die and most of them probably do so within the first 4–7 days after emigration from the marrow. Studies with [³H]-thymidine labelling *in vivo* have shown that both the T and the B cell pools in the periphery consist of short-lived, rapidly renewed cells and long-lived cells (6,7). These may correspond to primary and secondary (memory) cells, respectively. It is likely that those B cells which do not become

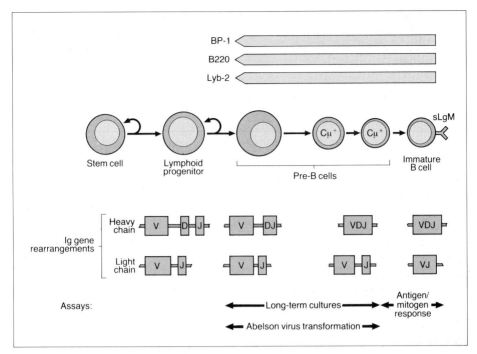

Figure 2.1.   Scheme of bone marrow B cell differentiation in the mouse. B cells develop from a putative common lymphoid progenitor cell. Shown are the recognizable stages of pre-B cell and early B cell development, together with key cell surface markers (shown at the top) Ig gene rearrangements and functional assays for B lineage cells.

activated by antigen die, whereas some of the progeny of those that are activated become long-lived B cells. Conceptually, this is an attractive mechanism for continuously renewing the potential antibody repertoire of the individual.

The factors which regulate B-lymphopoiesis are not well understood. What is known is that the rate of production is not regulated by end-cell feedback, unlike those of other marrow elements. Thus, treating mice with anti-μ antibodies during the neonatal period, which ablates the development of all B cells, does not affect the numbers of pre-B cells in the marrow (8). However, there is some evidence that bone marrow lymphocyte production is under the control of environmental influences. Firstly, it is reduced in germ-free mice. Secondly, production is increased by the injection of various foreign agents, such as sheep erythrocytes. This appears to be an antigen-non-specific phenomenon, which may be mediated by products of activated macrophages (cytokines?) in the spleen (9).

3.3 Culture systems for studying B cell development

Various systems have been devised for culturing B cell progenitors which have greatly helped in unravelling the various stages of B cell development. The classical Dexter long-term bone marrow culture system permits the differentiation of myeloid cells (principally granulocytes and macrophages), but not B cells. This was modified by Whitlock and Witte (10) to produce culture conditions that support B cell development. Another lymphoid culture system utilizes cells from fetal liver, but with a bone-marrow-derived feeder layer. The success of these culture systems depends on the presence of bone-marrow-derived stromal cells. Stromal cells are a heterogeneous population, since some cloned lines can support B cell differentiation whilst others cannot (11). How stromal cells provide the necessary micro-environment for B lymphopoiesis remains largely unknown. The intimate association between stromal cells and haematopoietic cells *in vivo* suggests that cell – cell contacts may be important. In addition, soluble growth factors similar to those acting on other haematopoietic lineages are undoubtedly also involved, some of which are produced by stromal cells. One of these has recently been gene cloned: it is a protein of M_r 25 kDa which has been named interleukin-7 (IL-7) (12), or more descriptively lymphopoietin-1. The molecule stimulates growth (but not differentiation) of B cell precursors which have not yet rearranged their Ig genes, and it also acts on immature thymocytes. It is therefore likely that a major target of IL-7 *in vivo* is the putative common lymphoid progenitor cell.

Immortalized lines of murine pre-B cells can be generated by transformation with the Abelson leukaemia virus, which have been widely used for studying the genetics of Ig gene rearrangements.

4. Ig gene rearrangements during B cell development

In the germline (or in non-B cells) the gene segments encoding V, D, J, and C segments discussed in Chapter 1 are separated from one another on the chromosome. As B cells develop from their progenitors these gene segments undergo an ordered series of recombination events to yield a functional sIgM molecule (13). The first event is the joining of a D segment to a J_H segment, closely followed by recombination with a particular V segment (*Figure 2.1*). The resulting pre-B cells now produce a complete μ chain. This is believed to prevent further V_H to DJ rearrangement in the cell and hence results in H-chain allelic exclusion. It apparently also induces the onset of L-chain V region gene rearrangements and the production of either kappa or lambda L-chains. Once the cells produce a complete IgM molecule this prevents further rearrangements in either the L- or H-chain V-region loci. In the mouse these immature sIgM[+] B cells can be detected by day 17 of fetal life.

4.1 V gene expression in the utilized repertoire

The V_H gene segments have been grouped into 10 families in the mouse, based on DNA or amino acid sequence similarities. Individual members of a particular family are, broadly speaking, clustered on the chromosome, although they are not strictly arranged in tandem. There is also evidence for V_H families in man. Studies of family-specific RNA in total extracts of fetal liver and of murine pre-B cell lines generated by immortalization with Abelson virus have indicated that there is preferential expression of J_H-proximal V_H families (i.e. 7183 and Q52) early in ontogeny (reviewed in 14). In adult tissues the representation of RNA specific for the various families more nearly approximates the actual distribution of the families. It is not known how this normalization of repertoire expression comes about. The frequency of B cells responsive to haptens such as DNP is similar in neonatal and adult mice. However, the numbers of distinct clonal precursors (clonotypes) are much smaller in neonatal animals, thereby indicating that the neonatal repertoire is severely restricted. There is evidence that these early clonotypes also preferentially use J-proximal V-regions (15).

4.2 Size of the utilized repertoire

As discussed in Chapter 1, the various genetic mechanisms involved in producing functional V-region genes could potentially generate some $10^8 - 10^9$ antibody specificities. Functional studies, however, indicate that the utilized repertoire is probably smaller than this. This problem has been studied by estimating the frequency of functional precursors and the number of clonotypes to a particular epitope using antigen- or mitogen-stimulated limiting dilution cultures. This approach has yielded a number of important conclusions about the mechanisms whereby the primary B cell repertoire is selected and regulated (13). Firstly, B cells responsive to haptens such as DNP or NIP occur at frequencies of $1:5000 - 1:10^4$ splenic B cells, while the number of different clonotypes is $c.$ 5000/hapten. These estimates therefore suggest that the utilized repertoire consists of $c.$ 10^7 specificities. Secondly, even with haptens which elicit restricted antibody responses, such as phosphorylcholine (PC) in Balb/c mice (where some 90% of the response consists of one clonotype called T15), precursor frequencies do not exceed $1/5 \times 10^4$ splenic B cells. Thirdly, environmental influences do not appear to affect diversification of the primary B cell repertoire. Analysis of the Balb/c anti-PC response, for example, indicates that the dominance of T15 is the result of non-random selection of V-region genes.

4.3 Expression of other sIg isotypes

All B cells initially express sIgM receptors. Most of the cells then also express sIgD, which first appears on mouse B cells around day 7 of neonatal life. In the adult, $c.$ 90% of splenic B cells express varying levels of both of these isotypes, although there is a small subpopulation which is sIgD-negative. Heavy-chain class switching to IgG, IgA, or IgE in antigen-stimulated B cells occurs by recombinations involving switch (S) regions upstream of the appropriate C-region genes (Chapter 3). However, co-expression of C_μ and C_δ (in association with a single V_H gene product) occurs without gene rearrangements since C_δ is not preceded by an S-region (16). It appears that these three gene segments form a single transcription unit which can give rise to μ or δ mRNAs by alternative RNA processing mechanisms, which are not understood in detail (*Figure 2.2*). Similar mechanisms of RNA processing later on determine whether a stimulated B cell will make surface or secreted IgM (Chapter 3).

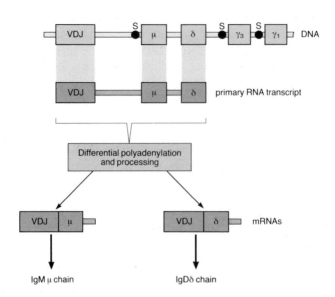

Figure 2.2.   Alternative RNA processing to yield sIgM and sIgD receptors. Shown at the top is part of the murine H-chain locus. All C genes apart from Cδ are preceded by switch sequences (S). The primary RNA transcript in most resting B cells runs from V_H, through Cμ and Cδ. The RNA is then processed to yield mRNA for either μ or δ chains (in association with the same rearranged V gene). Finally, the two H-chain proteins associate with a common pool of kappa or lambda L-chains.

The stage in B cell development at which cells start to express sIgG, sIgE, or sIgA is still a matter of debate. There is evidence from man, mouse, and chickens that this can occur early in ontogeny (presumably in the primary B cell repertoire), thereby generating cells which carry 3 classes of sIg (17). However, cells like these are quite rare in mammals, and most class switching to downstream isotypes is T cell controlled and occurs after activation of B cells by antigen (see Chapters 3 and 4).

5. B cell differentiation antigens

Apart from sIg receptors for antigen, B cells, like other cells, express a large array of cell membrane glycoproteins, some of which may be receptors for other ligands (such as cytokines), or which are involved in cell – cell interactions. The tracing of cell lineages by surface markers has been revolutionized by the advent of monoclonal antibodies (McAb). These have proved to be powerful tools for the analysis of complex mixtures of cells by multi-parametric flow cytometry, using the Fluorescence Activated Cell Sorter.

The antigens detected by the large number of McAb against human lymphocytes are periodically reviewed at International Workshops on Human Leucocyte Differentiation Antigens. These workshops have introduced the CD

Table 2.1. Major differentiation antigens of human B cells

Antigen[a]	B cell specific[b]	Nature[c]	Comments[d]
CD19	yes	gp95	Pan B
CD20	yes	p37/32	Pan B
CD21	no	p140	CR2
CD23	no	gp45–50	FcεRII
CDw32	no	gp40	FcγRII
CD35	no	gp250	CR1
CD40	no	gp50	
CD72	yes	gp43/39	Pan B

[a]CD designation (taken from 18)
[b]B cell specificity of the antigen
[c]Mol. weight of protein (gp = glycoprotein) in kDa
[d]Pan B = present on all B cells; otherwise refers to function of protein

Table 2.2. Major differentiation antigens of mouse B cells

Antigen[a]	B cell specific[b]	Nature[c]	Comments[d]
Ly-5(B220)	yes	p220	Pan B
Ly-17	no	p55–60	FcγRII (CD32)
Ly-42	yes?	p49	FcεRII (CD23)
Ly-44	yes	?	
Lyb-2	yes	p45	
Lyb-3	yes	?	B subset
Lyb-4	yes	?	
Lyb-5	yes	?	B subset
Lyb-6	yes	p45	
Lyb-7	yes	?	B subset
Lyb-8	yes	?	

[a]Accepted nomenclature (taken from 19)
[b]Specific for B cells
[c]Mol. weight of protein, if known
[d]Pan B = reactive with all B cells; B subset = reacts with a fraction of B cells. CD nomenclature given in parentheses

(cluster determinant) nomenclature, whereby antigens are defined on the basis of reactivity with a panel of McAb (reviewed in 18).

The major (more or less) B cell-specific antigens in mouse and man are summarized in *Table 2.1* and *Table 2.2*. These antigens are divided into molecules which are expressed on all B cells ('pan-B' markers) and those that are only present on a fraction of B cells. Some of the latter group occur on quiescent B cells, whereas others are activation antigens, expressed only when the cells have been stimulated in some way. It is evident that only a few of these antigens are specific for the B cell lineage. CD19 is the best B lineage marker in man, which appears on pre-B cells and which is retained on mature cells up to the plasma cell stage. CD24 is also expressed early during differentiation, but it is also present on polymorphs and some other cells. CD20 and CD37 react with all peripheral B cells, but not reliably with earlier differentiation stages.

The functions of some of these molecules are more or less understood. Examples are CD21 (= CR2) and CD35 (= CR1), which are receptors for split products of the C3 component of complement (see Chapter 4), and CDw32, which is one type of Fc receptor (FcRγII, see Chapter 4). Similarly, CD23 is a low-affinity FcR for IgE (FcεRII). In many cases, however, the most that is known about the antigen is its molecular weight.

The differentiation antigens on mouse lymphocytes are mostly designated by the 'Ly' (or in the case of B cells 'Lyb') nomenclature (reviewed in 19), although some of them clearly correspond to known CD antigens (*Table 2.2*). The best lineage marker is Ly-5(B220), which is the B cell version of the leukocyte common antigen (generically called CD45 in man): B220 is first expressed on pro-pre-B cells and is present on all peripheral B cells. Another marker called BP-1 is expressed early in B cell development, but then lost as cells mature through the pre-B cell compartment (see *Figure 2.1*). Although not shown in *Table 2.2*, all mouse B cells express CR1 and CR2.

In addition to these markers all B cells in both species carry Class I and Class II (Ia) MHC antigens. The importance of Class II molecules in TD B cell activation is discussed in Chapter 3. Finally, B cells also express a variety of surface molecules which are widely distributed on various cell types, such as CD11a/CD18 (leukocyte function antigen, LFA-1). This is also believed to be important in T cell – B cell interactions (see Chapter 3).

6. CD5 (Ly1)-positive B cells

The Ly1 antigen was originally described as a marker of helper T cells in the mouse. Subsequent analyses with monoclonal antibodies revealed that it is present on all mouse T cells, as is the human homologue CD5. CD5 is also found on a subpopulation of B cells in both species (representing about 1% of all murine B cells and 10 – 25% of peripheral blood B cells in man) with rather special properties (20,21). Phenotypically, the cells express high levels of sIgM and low levels of sIgD. In normal adult mice these cells constitute 20 – 40% of B cells in the peritoneal cavity, whilst they are rare in the spleen and effectively absent in lymph nodes. The levels of these cells are markedly elevated in some immunodefective strains of mice (such as the NZB and motheaten viable strains) and virtually absent in others (such as the CBA/N, see below). It is noteworthy that many B cell tumours, most notably B cell chronic lymphocytic leukaemias (B-CLL), appear to arise within the CD5$^+$ B cell population.

6.1 Origins

CD5$^+$ B cells constitute the majority of B cells in the human fetus and in the neonatal mouse. In the latter they are effectively replaced by ingress of 'conventional' B cells within a few weeks. CD5$^+$ cells develop originally from sIg-negative precursors in the bone marrow which seed the periphery in early life, although the relationship between them and the precursors of normal B cells is still unclear. However, in adult mice CD5$^+$ B cells constitute a self-renewing B cell subpopulation, clearly different from the conventional B cell pool. In other words, sIg-positive cells within the CD5$^+$ subpopulation are themselves capable of self-regeneration.

6.2 Repertoire

CD5$^+$ B cells produce much of the normal serum Ig (mostly IgM) in mice. Certain germline V_H and V_L genes are repeatedly and identically expressed in clonally unrelated CD5$^+$ B cells and these rarely undergo somatic mutations (22). These cells thus appear to express a limited repertoire of antibody specificities, including those for common environmental antigens such as phosphorylcholine (PC) and α1,3-dextran, and they also produce many autoantibodies. This is in line with the elevated levels of CD5$^+$ B cells found in autoimmune-prone strains of mice and in patients with rheumatoid arthritis (23). Antibody production by CD5$^+$ B cells appears to be T cell-independent: these B cells have not been shown to participate in classical TD antibody responses (see Chapter 3) nor to develop into memory cells.

6.3 Possible functions

The CD5$^+$ B cell compartment may be involved in natural immunity (24). This hypothesis envisages that (unknown) regulatory influences in early life lead to the selective expansion of clones expressing certain germline V-regions. There is evidence that the repertoire of early neonatal B cells contains many autoreactive specificities which are also multi-specific and interconnecting, that is, many of these antibodies are reactive with the combining sites (idiotypes) of other antibodies (25). The significance of anti-idiotypic reactivities within the immune system will be further discussed in Chapter 4. In the present context idiotype – anti-idiotype interactions during the neonatal period may be an important mechanism for shaping the developing repertoire, resulting in the selective expansion of clones expressing certain V-regions. These are then somehow 'imprinted' on the CD5$^+$ B cell pool and continually regenerated during the life of the individual (*Figure 2.3*). This is presumably because these V-regions have important survival value against common microbial pathogens. The high incidence of autoantibodies within the repertoire of CD5$^+$ B cells may therefore be because natural immunity is directed towards those microbial antigens which the pathogen cannot mutate: these would include epitopes which mimic host components, which micro-organisms have evolved during the process of host – parasite co-adaption.

In this scenario, the normal B cell population is therefore regarded as providing a *mutable* defence system, which adapts its responses to antigens which parasites can mutate. The evidence for antigen-driven hypermutation in antibodies is discussed in Chapter 4.

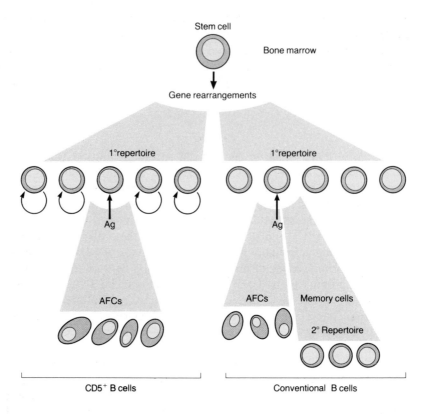

Figure 2.3. Postulated roles of CD5+ and 'conventional' B cells in immunity. As discussed in the text, both populations are originally bone-marrow derived. The CD5+ B cell repertoire is laid down in early life, and is then maintained by self-renewal by B cells in the periphery. Antigen (Ag) stimulates appropriate clones of cells to become AFC (but not memory cells). In contrast, the conventional B cell pool is continuously renewed from the bone marrow throughout life. Here stimulation with antigen elicits both AFC and memory cells: the latter have mutated their V-region genes to generate a secondary B cell repertoire, with higher affinity for the Ag (see Chapter 4).

7. Defects in B cell development

7.1 In man

A wide spectrum of clinical syndromes associated with defects in serum Ig levels (hypo- or agammaglobulinaemias), or antibody responses, has been described in man. Examples are X-linked agammaglobulinaemia, common variable hypogammaglobulinaemia, selective deficiencies of Ig isotypes or subclasses, Wiskott – Aldrich Syndrome, and ataxia-telangiectasia (reviewed in 26). The detailed pathogenesis of most of these conditions is still poorly understood, and only one of them is clearly a genetic defect in B cell development in the bone marrow. This is X-linked (Bruton's, or congenital) agammaglobulinaemia. Boys affected with this disease suffer severe infections, especially with encapsulated bacteria, after the age of 3–6 months. They exhibit an almost total absence of peripheral B cells, with normal levels of pre-B cells and of functional T cells. The μ-chains produced by the pre-B cells appear to be abnormal and have incomplete $V_H – D – J_H$ rearrangements. The condition may therefore result from a defect in an X-linked gene involved in VDJ recombination, although other explanations are possible.

7.2 In mice

The most widely studied murine model of humoral immunodeficiency is the CBA/N mouse, which carries an X-linked immunodeficiency (*xid*) (reviewed in 27). These mice have normal numbers of functional T cells, but have *c.* 50% fewer B cells than normal animals: the remaining B cells are phenotypically immature, expressing high levels of sIgM and low levels of sIgD. CBA/N mice have proven useful in defining two types of TI antigens (28). Their most striking immunological defect is an absolute failure to respond to long-chain poly-saccharide antigens, such as dextrans, pneumococcal capsular polysaccharides, and haptenated Ficoll (poly-sucrose) (called TI-2 antigens). Their B cells respond more normally to TI-1 antigens, as exemplified by haptenated or native lipopolysaccharide (LPS) and *Brucella abortus*. Their responses to various TD antigens (such as foreign erythrocytes or hapten–protein conjugates) are also more or less normal.

For several years it was believed that the phenotype of the CBA/N strain reflected the existence of two B cell subpopulations, with differential responsiveness to TI-1 and TI-2 antigens. This concept was supported by studies with polyclonal alloantisera which defined a differentiation antigen called Lyb-5. It appeared that Lyb-5$^-$ B cells respond to TI-1 and (with the aid of T_H cells) to TD antigens, whilst Lyb-5$^+$ cells (i.e. those absent in the CBA/N) respond to TI-2 antigens. Recent careful analyses have failed to provide convincing evidence in favour of this simple interpretation. The Lyb-5 antigen has remained elusive and attempts to raise monoclonal antibodies against it have uniformly failed. Secondly, B cells in CBA/N mice apparently express Lyb-5 following activation (29). An additional complication is that CBA/N mice lack CD5$^+$ B cells, which seem to play a major role in antibody responses against TI-2 antigens (30). The *xid* phenotype is therefore probably not due to the absence of a distinct B cell subpopulation, but rather a reflection of an (undefined) maturational arrest in the B cell pool.

The *xid* locus is tightly linked to a large gene family called XLR (X-linked, lymphocyte-regulated cluster), which is only transcribed in the later stages of B cell (and probably T cell) maturation (31). Certainly the fact that many animal and human immunodeficiencies follow an X-linked pattern of inheritance is evidence for the existence of genes on the X-chromosome which are crucially involved in controlling lymphocyte differentiation.

8. Further reading

Alt,F.W., Blackwell,T.K. and Yancopolous,G.D. (1987) *Science,* **238**, 1079.
Herzenberg,L.A., Stall,A.M., Lalor,P.A., Sidman,C.A., Moore,W.A., Parks,D.R. and
   Herzenberg,L.A. (1986) *Immunol. Rev.,* **93**, 81.
Osmond,D.G. (1986) *Immunol. Rev.,* **93**, 103.

9. References

1. Glick,B., Chang,T.S. and Jaap,R.G. (1956) *Poultry Sci.,* **35**, 224.
2. Reynaud,C.A., Anquez,V., Dahan,A. and Weill,J.C. (1985) *Cell,* **40**, 283.
3. Spangrude,G.J., Muller-Sieberg,C.E., Heimfeld,S. and Weissman,I.L. (1988) *J. Exp. Med.,* **167**, 1671.
4. Calvert,J.E. and Cooper,M.D. (1988) In *B Lymphocytes in Human Disease.* Bird,G. and Calvert,J.E. (ed.), Blackwell Scientific Publications, Oxford, p. 77.
5. Opstelten,D. and Osmond,D.G. (1983) *J. Immunol.,* **131**, 2635.
6. Press,O.W., Rosse,C. and Clagett,J. (1977) *Cell. Immunol.,* **33**, 114.
7. Freitas,A.A., Rocha,B. and Coutinho,A. (1986) *Immunol. Rev.,* **91**, 5.
8. Burrows,P.D., Kearney,J.F., Lawton,A.R. and Cooper,M.D. (1978) *J. Immunol.,* **120**, 1526.
9. Pietrangelli,C.E. and Osmond,D.G. (1985) *Cell. Immunol.,* **94**, 147.
10. Whitlock,C.A., Robertson,D. and Witte,O.N. (1984) *J. Immunol. Methods,* **67**, 353.
11. Kincade,P.W. (1989) *Ann. Rev. Immunol.,* **7**, 111.
12. Henney,C.S. (1989) *Immunol. Today,* **10**, 170.
13. Paige,C. and Wu,G.E. (1989) *FASEB J.,* **3**, 1818.
14. Alt,F.W., Blackwell,T.K., DePinho,R.A., Reth,M.G. and Yancopoulos,G.D. (1986) *Immunol. Rev.,* **89**, 5.
15. Klinman,N.R. and Linton,P.J. (1988) *Adv. Immunol.,* **42**, 1.
16. Yuan,D. and Tucker,P.W. (1984) *J. Exp. Med.,* **160**, 564.
17. Webb,C.F., Burrows,P.D., Borzillo,G.V. and Cooper,M.D. (1985) In *Monographs in Allergy: International Symposium on Ig Subclass Deficiencies.* Dukor,P., Kallos,P., Trnka,Z. and Waksman,B.H. (ed.), Karger, Basle, p. 1.
18. Knapp,W., Rieber,P., Dorken,B., Schmidt,R.E., Stein,H. and van den Borne,A.E.G. (1989) *Immunol. Today,* **10**, 253.
19. Holmes,K.L. and Morse,H.C. (1988) *Immunol. Today,* **9**, 344.
20. Caligaris-Cappio,F., Gobbi,M., Bofill,M. and Janossy,G. (1982) *J. Exp. Med.,* **155**, 623.
21. Hayakawa,K., Hardy,R.R., Parks,D.R. and Herzenberg,L.A. (1983) *J. Exp. Med.,* **157**, 202.
22. Forster,I., Gu,H. and Rajewsky,K. (1988) *EMBO J.,* **7**, 3693.
23. Plater-Zyberk,C., Maini,R.N., Lam,K., Kennedy,T.D. and Janossy,G. (1985) *Arthritis Rheum.,* **28**, 971.
24. Kocks,C. and Rajewsky,K. (1989) *Ann. Rev. Immunol.,* **7**, 537.
25. Vakil,M. and Kearney,J.F. (1986) *Eur. J. Immunol.,* **16**, 1151.
26. Bird,G. (1988) In *B Lymphocytes in Human Disease.* Bird,G. and Calvert,J.E. (ed.), Oxford University Press, Oxford, p. 257.
27. Scher,I. (1982) *Adv. Immunol.,* **33**, 2.
28. Mosier,D.E., Scher,I. and Paul,W.E. (1976) *J. Immunol.,* **117**, 1363.
29. Smith,H.R., Yaffe,L.J., Kastner,D.L. and Steinberg,A.D. (1986) *J. Immunol.,* **136**, 1194.
30. Hayakawa,K., Hardy,R.R. and Herzenberg,L.A. (1986) *Eur. J. Immunol.,* **16**, 450.
31. Cohen,D.I., Steinberg,A.D., Paul,W.E. and Davis,M.M. (1985) *Nature,* **314**, 372.

3

B cell activation: induction of
the primary antibody response

1. Introduction

In a normal healthy individual most lymphocytes in the periphery are quiescent cells, that is, in G_0. Upon encountering antigen, clones of either T and/or B cells are activated, enter cell cycle, and differentiate into effector cells and/or memory cells. In this chapter we will consider the events which control the development of B cells into AFC, which produce the primary antibody response. The production of AFC and memory cells (see Chapter 4) are regulated by a combination of cell – cell interactions and soluble growth and differentiation factors (cytokines), many of which are secreted by T_H cells.

2. Polyclonal B cell activation

Before considering specific antibody responses it is necessary to discuss the properties of agents which stimulate lymphocytes polyclonally, that is, irrespective of their antigen specificities (*Figure 3.1*). Polyclonal activators (also called T or B cell mitogens) mimic, at least some of, the effects of specific antigens on lymphocytes. Some of them primarily activate T cells (e.g. concanavalin A or phytohaemagglutinin), whilst others principally affect B cells (*Table 3.1*). These agents are therefore invaluable for studies of the biochemistry and molecular biology of lymphocyte activation. Some polyclonal activators only induce B cells to proliferate, whilst others also stimulate secretion of Ig with a broad range of specificities as well.

2.1 Activators of human B cells

These include lectins such as pokeweed mitogen, agents which cross-link sIg receptors (anti-Ig antibodies and *Staph. aureus Cowan*), as well as Epstein – Barr virus (EBV), the causative agent of infectious mononucleosis and Burkitt's

Specific antigen	Polyclonal activator

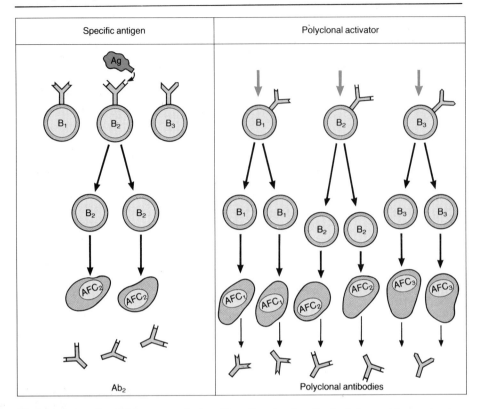

Figure 3.1.   Specific versus polyclonal B cell activation. In the left panel immunization with Ag leads to the activation of Ag-specific clones of B cells (shown as B2) which ultimately become AFC secreting antibodies specific for that antigen. In the right panel stimulation with a polyclonal activator (such as LPS) causes activation of clones with many different specificities (B1, 2, and 3), thereby leading to the secretion of antibodies reactive with a variety of different epitopes.

lymphoma. The induction of antibody secretion by all these agents is T cell-dependent, with the exception of EBV. EBV is a rather special case: it acts as a true TI polyclonal B cell activator, provoking the secretion of IgM, IgG, and IgA. However, the virus can also transform human B cells, producing immortalized B cell lines. EBV binds to the CR2 (CD21) receptor, which is physiologically important in the control of B cell activation (see Chapter 4).

Monoclonal antibodies to a variety of human B cell markers also induce B cell activation, either on their own or together with co-stimuli, such as phorbol myristic acetate (PMA) or cytokines. These McAb have attracted considerable interest because the cell surface proteins may be important physiological regulators of B cell activation. Examples are CD20, CD23, CD21, and CD40 (reviewed in 1). CD20 is a particularly interesting molecule since it has been shown to be a Ca^{2+} channel. CD23 (FcεRII) is a marker of activated B cells: a cleaved form of this molecule acts as an autocrine growth factor for human B cells and it is likely that CD23 is intimately involved in the regulation of IgE responses.

Table 3.1. Polyclonal B cell activators

Agent	T-dependent	Ig secretion
a For human B cells		
Pokeweed mitogen	yes	yes
Staph. aureus Cowan	yes	yes
LPS	yes?	yes
Epstein – Barr virus[a]	no	yes
Anti-Ig	no	no[b]
b For mouse B cells		
LPS	no	yes
Pokeweed mitogen	yes	yes
PPD[c]	no	yes
Anti-Ig	no	no[b]

[a]Also causes transformation of human B cells
[b]Can stimulate Ig secretion in the presence of cytokines
[c]Purified protein derivative of tuberculin

2.2 Activators of mouse B cells

The commonest activators used with mouse B cells are LPS, and anti-Ig antibodies (*Table 3.1*). LPS is a powerful activator, which stimulates both DNA synthesis and polyclonal Ig secretion in some 10 – 30% of splenic B cells. There are also McAb which stimulate murine B cells; for example, those directed against Lyb-2 (2).

2.3 Stimulation of B cells by anti-Ig

Anti-Ig antibodies are particularly attractive B cell activators since they will hopefully mimic the effects of antigen binding to sIg receptors. High concentrations of purified rabbit or goat anti-Ig antibodies—generally F(ab')$_2$ fragments of anti-μ, anti-δ, or anti-L chain—induce all mouse B cells to become activated (see below) and up to 30% to progress to DNA synthesis. Anti-Ig does not induce Ig secretion, except in the presence of cytokines (reviewed in 3). Lower concentrations of anti-Ig induce resting B cells to become abortively activated (see below), but not to synthesize DNA (*Figure 3.2*). The mitogenicity of anti-Ig is markedly enhanced by co-culturing B cells with cytokines, especially IL-4 (see Section 4.4.1). Studies with monoclonal anti-Ig have shown that extensive cross-linking of sIg receptors is needed for optimal B cell activation by this route. In line with this, the mitogenic potency of anti-Ig is greatly enhanced by coupling the antibodies to agarose beads, or to long-chain polymers such as dextran (4). It is therefore likely that anti-Ig stimulation represents a polyclonal model for B cell activation by bacterial TI-2 antigens (see Section 5).

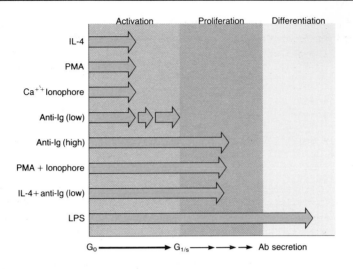

Figure 3.2. Examples of polyclonal activators for mouse B cells which cause different degrees of stimulation. Certain agents (such as IL-4, low concentrations of anti-Ig) only cause resting B cells to become activated, but not to proliferate. Often two of these abortive activators can synergize with each other to induce B cells to synthesize DNA (e.g. IL-4 plus a low concentration of anti-Ig). Of the agents shown, only LPS induces B cells to mature into AFC.

2.3.1 Signal transduction by sIg receptors

The use of anti-Ig has yielded much information about the second messengers utilized by sIg receptors. Both sIgM and sIgD receptors on B cells are typical Ca^{2+}-mobilizing receptors (reviewed in 5). Ligation of sIg stimulates the breakdown of phosphatidylinositol 4,5 bisphosphate in the cell membrane, yielding two intracellular second messengers: inositol 1,4,5 trisphosphate, which mobilizes Ca^{2+} from intracellular stores, and 1,2 diacylglycerol, which is an essential co-factor for the key regulatory enzyme protein kinase C (PKC). This signalling cascade is controlled by an uncharacterized guanine-nucleotide binding (G) protein, which couples sIg receptors to the phospholipase C (6). Both the Ca^{2+} signal and PKC activation are required to achieve optimal B cell activation via this pathway (*Figure 3.2*): mouse B cells synthesize DNA when cultured with a Ca^{2+} ionophore (which increases intracellular Ca^{2+} levels) plus a PKC activator such as PMA, but not in response to either agent alone (7).

Other polyclonal B cell activators, such as LPS, do not induce Ca^{2+} mobilization, thereby indicating that there are multiple pathways for activating resting B cells (8).

3. Stages in primary B cell stimulation

It has become traditional to divide the events which follow the activation of quiescent B cells (by specific antigen or by a polyclonal stimulus) into three stages:

activation, proliferation, and differentiation (*Figure 3.2*). Thus division is convenient for descriptive and experimental purposes. However, in reality it is artificial since, for example, the genetic programme for the induction of antibody secretion in LPS-stimulated B cells is gradually turned on as the cells undergo successive rounds of division.

3.1 Activation

This refers to the events which occur in the first 24 h following stimulation of small, quiescent B cells, and which precede the entry of the cells into the G_1 phase of the cell cycle. The earliest changes which occur in this period are the generation of the intracellular second messengers mentioned above, and the appearance of mRNA for products of cellular oncogenes such as *c-fos* and *c-myc* (9). The cells gradually enlarge: changes in cell surface markers also occur during this period, such as increases in the levels of CD23 and Ia antigens (1). The increase in MHC Class II expression is undoubtedly of major importance for the subsequent interaction of the B cell with an appropriate T_H cell (see Section 4.2). A variety of agents (low concentrations of anti-Ig, IL-4, Ca^{2+} ionophores, and PMA) induce B cells to enter this 'poised' activation state (*Figure 3.2*). Cells cultured with such 'abortive activators' will only synthesize DNA if they receive additional stimuli.

3.2 Growth or proliferation

This refers to the entry of activated (blast) cells into the G_1 phase of their first cycle (heralded by the onset of increasing rates of RNA and protein synthesis) and their eventual commitment to DNA synthesis and one or more rounds of cell division. The physiological purpose of this phase is obviously to expand rapidly the numbers of antigen-reactive cells capable of producing antibodies to the priming antigen. During the induction of a specific antibody response this phase, and the concomitant differentiation of these B cell blasts into AFC, is controlled by cytokines released by T_H cells (see Section 4.4).

3.3 Differentiation to AFC

Much of the available information about this phase has emerged from extensive studies of LPS-activated murine B cells. B cells cultured with LPS start to secrete IgM after some 30 h and the levels produced by individual cells continue to increase over the next few days. Differentiation is accompanied by marked morphological changes: early AFC are large lymphoblasts, and these gradually mature into typical plasma cells, with extensive lamellar endoplasmic reticulum (10). Plasma cells are highly differentiated end-cells, with a lifespan of only a few days: 5–40% of their protein synthesis is devoted to antibody production (see *Figure 1.1*).

3.3.1 The induction of IgM secretion

Activated primary B cells initially secrete IgM antibodies. The H and L chains are synthesized and combine in the endoplasmic reticulum, the H chains are

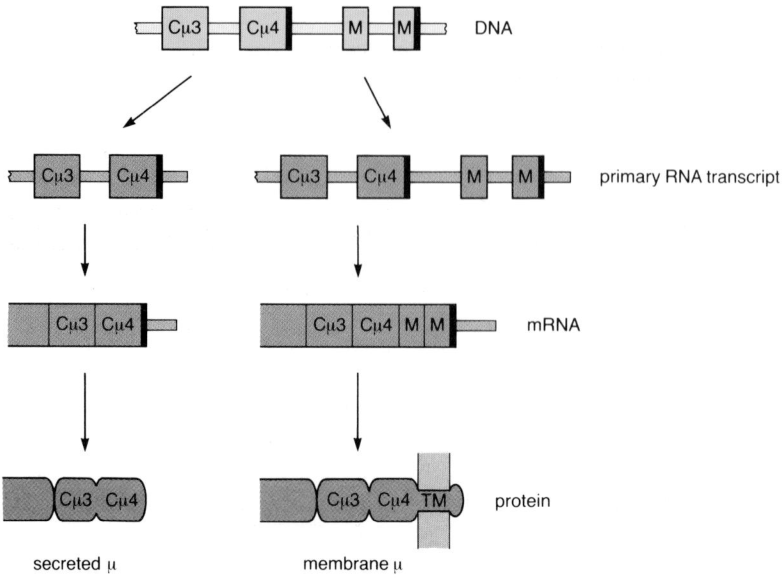

Figure 3.3.   Alternative RNA processing to yield the membrane or secreted forms of the μ H-chain. At the top are shown the two C-terminal exons (Cμ3 and 4) and two M exons which generate the transmembrane (TM) segment. Both Cμ4 and M2 have a stop sequence (black bars) at their 3' end. These can therefore yield two primary transcripts and two mRNA species. If transcription stops after Cμ4 the transcript with a polyA tail is processed to produce mRNA for μs. If transcription runs through M1 and M2 the terminal amino acids of Cμ4 and its associated S are removed by processing, and this leads to production of the μm protein.

glycosylated and the assembled protein is secreted by reverse pinocytosis from the Golgi complex. The C-terminal sequences of the H chains of membrane (m) and secreted (s) forms of IgM (and other isotypes) are structurally different: the μm form contains a hydrophobic transmembrane region and three intracytoplasmic residues, whilst the μs chain ends with a hydrophilic C-terminus. These two H-chains are translated from distinct mRNA molecules, because the rearranged μ gene consists of a complex transcription unit with multiple polyadenylation sites (*Figure 3.3*). The hydrophilic C-terminus of the μs chain is encoded as part of the Cμ4 domain, whilst the transmembrane region of μm is encoded by two separate M exons. Thus, in resting B cells, which only produce membrane IgM, RNA splicing joins the M exons directly to the end of Cμ4 exon, excluding the sequences for the C-terminus of μs. In activated B cells addition of poly(A) to the C-terminus of the Cμ4 exon is followed by RNA splicing to yield a secreted μ-chain (11,12). Similar alternative RNA processing controls the later expression of the surface or secreted forms of other isotypes.

3.3.2 Isotype switching

As mentioned in Chapter 2, switching to other isotypes at the level of sIg expression occurs to a limited extent in B cells soon after their emergence from

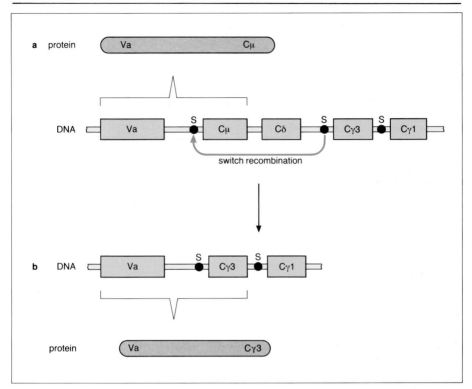

Figure 3.4. Switch recombination. **a** depicts a rearranged V gene (Va) which is transcribed together with Cμ in an IgM-secreting cell. There is a switch (S) sequence immediately upstream of each C_H gene (apart from Cδ). **b** During class switching, looping out and deletion of intervening DNA sequences thus lead to the transcription of Va together with (in this example) the Cγ3 gene.

the bone marrow, that is, in the apparent absence of antigen stimulation. For many years it was uncertain if antigen (or mitogen) driven IgG (IgA, IgE) responses are the result of intraclonal switching. This issue was resolved by the use of limiting dilution cultures, stimulated with mitogens such as LPS. Up to 80% of LPS-induced IgM-secreting clones switch to IgG production: the predominant isotypes are generally those encoded by C-region genes immediately downstream from Cμ and Cδ. Thus, IgG3 and IgG2b are found often, whilst IgA and IgE are quite rare (13,14). Switching to IgG requires several rounds of cell division (15).

Switching occurs via two mechanisms. The first, called switch recombination, involves the deletion of C_H genes 5′ to the expressed C_H gene (*Figure 3.4*) and its expression together with the complete V_H gene (16). However, switching can also occur in the absence of gene deletion. This presumably involves post-transcriptional processing of long nuclear RNA transcripts, in a similar manner to that described for the dual expression of sIgM and sIgD (Chapter 2). It is probable that this mechanism precedes switch recombination, which may only occur at the plasma cell stage. The resulting clonal progeny could therefore

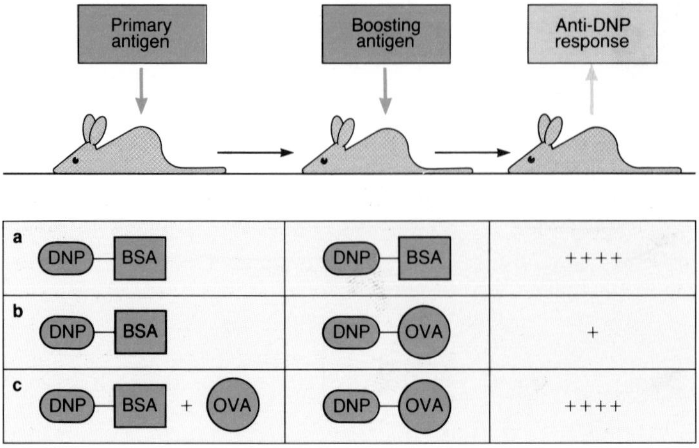

	Primary antigen	Boosting antigen	Anti-DNP response
a	DNP—BSA	DNP—BSA	++++
b	DNP—BSA	DNP—OVA	+
c	DNP—BSA + OVA	DNP—OVA	++++

Figure 3.5.   The carrier effect. In groups **a** and **b** mice were primarily immunized with DNP-bovine serum albumin (BSA) in adjuvant. Only those boosted with DNP-BSA make a substantial secondary anti-DNP antibody response, whereas those boosted with DNP on another carrier (ovalbumin, OVA) do not. In **c** mice were first immunized with OVA plus DNP-BSA, inducing the activation of OVA-specific T_H cells, so that these animals give a large secondary response to DNP-OVA.

express say both (secreted and membrane) IgM and IgG. IgM-secreting clones can also co-express two or, rarely, more isotypes of sIg. Thus, IgG3-secreting cells are likely to also express sIgG3 on their surfaces.

The fact that LPS *per se* can induce switching indicates that B cells have an inherent capacity to switch to downstream isotypes. However, as discussed below, switching during antibody responses to TD antigens is dramatically affected by T cells.

4. TD antibody formation

4.1 Introduction

The induction of antibody responses to most antigens requires the participation of both T_H cells and antigen-presenting cells (APC). The first evidence for T cell – B cell co-operation came from the work of Claman *et al.* in 1966 (17). They showed that irradiated mice could only make antibodies to sheep red blood cells (SRBC) if they were given both bone marrow and thymus cells. It rapidly became clear that although B cells produce the antibody response, they only do so with the help of thymus-derived T cells.

Another important milestone in the elucidation of the nature of cell co-operation came from studies on the so-called carrier effect (*Figure 3.5*). Small molecules (haptens) such as DNP only induce antibodies if they are coupled to an immunogenic (carrier) protein or cell. Mice immunized with DNP-carrier A make primary anti-DNP and anti-A antibody responses. However, these animals do not make a secondary (i.e. memory) anti-DNP response if challenged with

DNP on carrier B, unless they had also been immunized with B. Mitchison and others showed that the elicitation of a secondary anti-DNP response to DNP-carrier B in irradiated mice requires DNP-specific B memory cells and carrier B-immunized T_H cells (18,19).

These experiments provided the first clear evidence for co-operation of T and B cells with distinct epitopic specificities. They also indicated that hapten and carrier determinants must be physically linked on the same molecule. The experiments were interpreted as follows: B cells recognize DNP epitopes on the native hapten – carrier complex via their sIg receptors, whilst T cells recognize epitopes of the carrier protein via their antigen receptors. Co-operation was believed to result from the formation of an *antigen bridge* between the two cell types. This led to the delivery of (undefined) helper signals from the T cell to the B cell, thereby resulting in its activation to antibody secretion. This model has now been revised because of the realization that T cells do not recognize native proteins (see below). However, the concept that T_H cells and B cells interact physically during immune induction has stood the test of time (see Section 4.3.2).

The development of *in vitro* culture systems permitted the further dissection of the cellular interactions involved in the initiation of antibody responses. These led to the demonstration that highly purified T and B cells alone cannot respond to antigens such as SRBC. A third cell type is often required, which in this case was the macrophage (20), which processes and presents the antigen to the T cell (see below).

4.2 MHC-restricted (cognate) and unrestricted T cell help

The antigen-specific TCR on T cells only recognizes foreign antigens in association with self-MHC antigens (Class I or Class II molecules), a phenomenon known as MHC restriction. CD4-positive T_H cells recognize antigens in association with Class II antigens, whilst CD8-positive cytotoxic T cells require antigens to be presented in association with Class I antigens on APC. Both types of T cells only recognize antigens which have been denatured and, in many cases, cleaved by proteases in APC (*processed antigen*). The recent crystallographic resolution of the structure of a human Class I MHC protein (21) has provided a simple and graphic explanation for MHC restriction. These studies have suggested that peptides generated by APC bind to a groove in the MHC antigen. The V-regions of the appropriate TCR therefore bind to both the bound peptide and to surrounding regions of the MHC antigen.

The induction of TD antibody responses, especially those elicited from quiescent B cells, is MHC-restricted (e.g. 22,23). In other words, T_H cells and APC (and/or B cells) need to be from individuals which are compatible at the I-region in the mouse. For some time it was uncertain whether MHC restriction in antibody responses operates at the level of APC – T cell interaction, and/or at the level of T/B co-operation. This controversy was resolved by the demonstration that the requirements for the stimulation of resting B cells and pre-activated B cells differ markedly: resting B cells require MHC-restricted, cell – cell contact for activation. This is called *cognate help* (see below). In contrast, activated B cell blasts can be further stimulated by non-antigen specific growth and differentiation factors (*non-cognate, or factor-mediated help*: see Section 4.4). In addition, it has emerged that B cells themselves are very effective APC for the activation of T_H cells.

4.3 Cognate T cell – B cell interactions

4.3.1 B cells as APC

The major cell types which function as APC in lymphoid tissues are macrophages, dendritic cells, and B cells. These cells take up protein antigens, process them (usually to small peptides), and express the peptide fragments on their Class II molecules. The importance of B cells as APC was only recognized relatively recently. This is because it is difficult to prepare B cells absolutely free of macrophages and/or dendritic cells, which would complicate the assay system. This problem was neatly circumvented, initially by Chesnut and Grey (24), by using rabbit anti-mouse Ig (RaMIg) as an antigen. They compared the capacities of macrophages and B cells to present RaMIg, or normal rabbit IgG (RGG) to RGG-specific T cell clones. The results showed that the two cell types present RaMIg equally well to T cells, especially at low concentrations of antigen. However, B cells are much less efficient at presenting RGG to T cells. The explanation for these findings lies in the capacity of RaMIg to bind to sIg receptors on all B cells. B cells can therefore effectively concentrate antigens which bind to their sIg receptors and are then subsequently internalized and processed. In contrast, other proteins (such as RGG) are taken up rather poorly by B cells by fluid phase pinocytosis, a process which is much more efficient in macrophages. B cells present RaMIg to T cells at 10 000-fold lower protein concentrations than RGG, when only a fraction of the sIg receptors are occupied by antigen. B cells therefore act as immunological 'vacuum cleaners' to concentrate specific antigens. A particularly elegant demonstration of their capacity to act as APC came from a study by Lanzavecchia (25). He showed that human B cell clones (immortalized with EBV) specific for tetanus toxoid could very effectively present this protein to cloned antigen-specific T cells. This result provided definitive evidence that T cells and B cells can co-operate in the absence of macrophages or other types of APC.

The current consensus is therefore that B cells are indeed physiologically important APC for the activation of T_H cells. *In vivo* probably only those B cells with sIg receptors specific for the antigen are relevant, since only these will be able to take up and process sufficient antigen. Evidence for the importance of B cells as APC *in vivo* has come from experiments where mice were treated with anti-μ antibodies from birth, to ablate the development of B cells: this markedly suppresses the activation of T cells by protein antigens in lymph nodes (26).

The contemporary explanation for the hapten-carrier effect and linked recognition is therefore as follows (*Figure 3.6*). B cells recognizing haptenic moieties on the antigen concentrate and internalize it, process, and finally present peptide fragments of the complex on their Class II antigens to carrier-specific

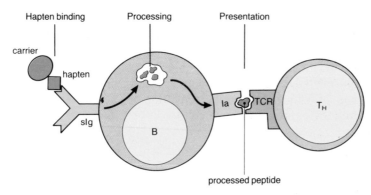

Figure 3.6. Current explanation for the carrier effect. A hapten-specific B cell binds a hapten – carrier complex via its sIg receptors. This cell internalizes and processes the antigen and finally presents carrier-derived peptides on its MHC Class II molecules to an appropriate T_H cell. This results in activation of the T cell and, in consequence, the B cell.

T cells. This leads to establishment of cell – cell contacts (see below), activation of the T cell, which then delivers helper signals to the B cell. This model does not exclude the initial activation of resting T cells by carrier-derived peptides expressed on other types of APC and their subsequent interaction with hapten-specific B cells.

It is worth mentioning here that other receptors apart from sIg may also mediate antigen uptake by B cells, in particular the FcR, CR1, and CR2. However, these are more likely to be involved during later phases of the response once circulating antibodies, and hence antigen – antibody complexes, have been formed. The role of these receptors in B cell responses is therefore considered in Chapter 4.

4.3.2 MHC-restricted conjugation between T and B cells

Activation of resting B cells by T_H cells requires physical contact between the two cell types. This conjugate formation has been studied in various model systems using T cell lines and antigen-specific B cells (27,28). The formation of stable tight unions requires specific antigen, B cells bearing the correct Class II protein, and a period of time for them to process the antigen. Under these conditions conjugation occurs within some 15 min, and the conjugates last for several hours. Conjugation is monogamous, that is, in general one T cell only binds one B cell, for unknown reasons. The interaction leads to the formation of areas of intimate membrane contact between the two cells, and a striking re-orientation of the microtubular organizing centre in the T cell towards the area of the cell contact (29). This is an intriguing observation, since this complex may promote the vectorial release of cytokines towards the attached B cell by directing secretory vesicles from the Golgi apparatus to the area of cell contact. Conjugate formation can be blocked by monoclonal antibodies against a variety of cell surface molecules on either cell type. These include the TCR, Thy-1, CD4, and LFA-1 on the T cell, and sIg, LFA-1, and Class II on the B cell.

It is therefore highly likely that these conjugates initially form as a result of T cell recognition of peptide fragments of antigen processed and expressed on the Class II molecules of the B cells. The conjugate is then further stabilized by cell adhesion molecules, including LFA-1 (a member of the integrin family of proteins) and CD4, which binds to Class II molecules. The biological consequences of conjugation can be activation of one or both partners, the T cell to secrete cytokines and the B cell to differentiate into AFC.

4.3.3 Signal transduction during cell – cell contact

It is still unclear what roles the various cell surface molecules known to be involved in stabilizing T-cell – B-cell conjugates play in inducing B cell activation. Two B cell molecules which are of potential importance are sIg and Class II. As discussed in Section 2.3 anti-Ig antibodies are powerful B cell activators. However, typical TD protein antigens do not cause substantial B cell activation in the absence of T cells (30). This is probably because most proteins do not carry sufficient numbers of repeating epitopes to extensively cross-link sIg. Even if the antigen can cause some cross-linking of sIg it is likely that the concentrations attained *in vivo* would only cause abortive B cell activation (see Section 3.1). This may be important, however, if it leads to an increase in Ia antigen levels on the B cell, which favours cell – cell interactions. In addition, if the interacting T cell secretes IL-4, this could synergize with antigen-induced signals to drive B cells into cycle (Section 3.1).

The precise role of Class II in B cell activation is controversial. Anti-Class II monoclonal antibodies can inhibit mitogen-induced B cell responses (31). On the other hand, there is evidence that Class II molecules can transduce stimulatory signals (32). Anti-Ia antibodies induce rises in cyclic AMP levels in mouse B cells, and also induce translocation of the key regulatory enzyme PKC (see Section 2.3) to the nucleus (33). The physiological significance of this remains to be established.

A major problem with studies using McAb against cell interaction molecules is that they may not accurately mimic the situation occurring during T-cell – B-cell conjugation. It is likely that the combined signals generated by the interactions between the various cell surface molecules known to be involved in conjugation determine the biological outcome of the union. In addition, soluble factors released at high concentrations into the area of cell – cell contact may also be important. Nevertheless, it is clear that a (currently undefined) cell-contact-mediated signal is an essential component of cognate help for resting B cells.

4.4 Non-cognate help: B cell cytokines

The growth and differentiation of large, pre-activated B cells can be stimulated by allogeneic T cells or their soluble products. These factors were originally identified as activities secreted by stimulated T cells, which replace T cells in the induction of TD antibody responses (T-cell-replacing factors, TRF). Further

Table 3.2.   Major cytokines with effects on B cells

Cytokine	Activation	Growth	Ig secretion
IL-1[a]		+	+
IL-2		+	+
IL-4[b]	+	+	+
IL-5[c]		+	+
IL-6		+	+
IFN$_\gamma$[d]	(+)	+	+

[a]Generally synergizes with other agents
[b]Causes growth with other stimuli; selective switching to IgG1 (in mouse) and IgE
[c]Clear effects in mouse B cells; uncertain in human
[d]Antagonizes many effects of IL-4 in mouse and man; selective production of IgG2a in mouse

characterization of these activities showed that some molecules act as B cell growth factors (BCGF), some induce differentiation of pre-activated cells to Ig secretion (BCDF activity), whilst others have both activities (B-cell-stimulating factors, BSF). These and other T cell (and in some cases macrophage) products are now generically called cytokines, lymphokines, or interleukins. At the time of writing, the genes for at least 8 interleukins have been cloned, and a considerable number of them, as well as other soluble molecules, have been shown to modulate B cell responses in a variety of *in vitro* assay systems (*Table 3.2*; reviewed in 34).

It should be stressed that the precise details of how these numerous factors control the various phases of B cell responses are not yet known. There are many reasons for the continuing state of confusion in this field. One major problem is that all cytokines are pleiotropic, and their activities are often not even specific for a particular haematopoietic cell lineage. In the present context, the demonstration that a particular cytokine is active in *in vitro* B cell assays does not necessarily mean that this activity reflects the pre-eminent physiological role of that molecule *in vivo*. In short, the best that one can therefore achieve at present is to catalogue the biological properties of those cytokines most likely to play an imporant role in antibody responses, and then to draw a (very speculative) synthesis, which will probably prove to be incorrect!

4.4.1 Interleukin-4 (BSF-1)

This T cell product could be important both during B cell activation and later on as a BCDF. It was first recognized by its capacity to synergize with non-mitogenic concentrations of anti-Ig to induce resting B cells to synthesize DNA (35; *Figure 3.2*). On its own IL-4 is an abortive activator (see Section 3.1), causing marked increases in Ia antigen and CD23 levels on B cells. It also promotes the production of IgG1 and IgE antibodies by B cells activated with LPS (36,37). There is little doubt that IL-4 plays a major role in the induction of IgE responses *in vivo* (38). IL-4 is a good example of a pleiotropic lymphokine, receptors for which are widely expressed on cells of various haematopoietic lineages. It is therefore not surprising that the factor exerts biological effects on many different cells, including mast cells, macrophages, and T cells (reviewed in 39).

4.4.2 Interleukin-5 (BCGF II)

IL-5 is also a T cell product, which acts as a BCGF and BCDF in *pre-activated* mouse B cells. In this species it is a major TRF, although probably not the only one (40). IL-5 promotes the production of IgM and IgG antibodies and also selectively enhances IgA production by LPS-activated B cells (41). Curiously, it has been rather difficult to demonstrate substantially similar effects of IL-5 on human B cells (42). This molecule is also not B cell-specific, since it stimulates the differentiation of eosinophils from precursor cells (43), and also acts on T cells.

4.4.3 Interleukin-6 (BSF-2)

This factor is produced by an extraordinarily wide array of cells, including T cells and macrophages (reviewed in 44). Its principal effect on human B cells is as a BCDF (but not BCGF) for pre-activated B cells and B cell lines. It also promotes the growth of factor-dependent hybridoma and plasmacytoma cell lines. It is a very pleiotropic molecule which (like IL-1) seems to play a major role in inflammation, since it promotes fever and acute-phase protein release by hepatocytes, besides exerting a wide variety of effects on the immune and haematopoietic systems.

4.4.4 Interleukin-2

This T cell product was initially recognized by its capacity to maintain the long-term growth of T cells. T cells only express high affinity IL-2 receptors following activation. Similarly, activated B cells can also express these receptors and can be induced to both proliferate and to secrete Ig by IL-2 (45,46). The evidence for this is clearer in human than in murine B cells, where it remains possible that only a subset of B cells can be induced to express functional IL-2 receptors by certain stimuli. A recent study indicates that IL-4 and IL-5 synergize to promote the expression of functional high-affinity IL-2 receptors in murine B cells (47).

4.4.5 Gamma Interferon (IFN_γ)

This T-cell product has both anti-viral and anti-proliferative activities and plays multiple roles in immune responses. It acts as a BCDF, especially for the induction of IgG2a antibody production in the mouse (48). A major effect of IFN_γ is to antagonize the effects of IL-4 in a variety of different assay systems (e.g. 49).

4.5 *T_H cell subsets producing different lymphokines*

Long-term antigen-specific murine CD4-positive T_H cell clones can be divided into two functional subpopulations according to the lymphokines which they

Table 3.3. Lymphokines produced by murine CD4$^+$ T cell subsets

Lymphokine	T_{H1}	T_{H2}
IFN$_\gamma$	+ +	–
IL-2	+ +	–
IL-3	+ +	+ +
IL-4	–	+ +
IL-5	–	+ +
IL-6	–	+ +
LT[a]	+ +	–
TNF[b]	+ +	+
GM-CSF[c]	+ +	+

[a]Lymphotoxin
[b]Tumour necrosis factor
[c]Granulocyte-macrophage colony-stimulating factor
(From Mosmann and Coffman, 1989)

secrete following stimulation by antigen (reviewed in 50). These are called T_{H1} and T_{H2} and their products are listed in *Table 3.3*. It is evident that some cytokines (such as IL-3) are produced by both types of T cell clone. The major differences between the two subsets is in their capacity to produce IL-2, IFN$_\gamma$ (T_{H1} cells), IL-4, IL-5, and IL-6 (T_{H2} cells).

Both T_{H1} and T_{H2} cells can help B cells to make antibodies. However, T_{H2} cells are generally more effective helpers than T_{H1} cells, especially for IgG1 and IgE responses. This is because they produce IL-4. Some T_{H1} clones can also provide help, but these favour the production of other isotypes such as IgG2a (probably as a result of IFN$_\gamma$ production, 48). A major function of T_{H1} cells is believed to be in mediating inflammatory responses, such as DTH reactions.

It is still uncertain to what extent this specialization in T_H cell function occurs *in vivo*. It is also unclear if T_{H1} and T_{H2} cells represent products of separate lineages, or whether they are different stages of one lineage. Currently available evidence favours the latter possibility.

4.5.1 Regulation of isotype production by lymphokines

Switching from initial IgM production to other isotypes (see Section 3.3.2) is markedly affected by T cells. Furthermore, individual cytokines have strikingly different effects on the production of different isotypes: for example, low doses of IL-4 suppress IgG3 secretion in LPS-stimulated B cells and promote both membrane expression and secretion of IgG1. Higher concentrations of IL-4 markedly stimulate the production of IgE (29,30). Similarly, IL-5 promotes the secretion of IgA, and IFN$_\gamma$ promotes the production of IgG2a. The effects of IL-4 reflect true lymphokine-directed switching, rather than the selective survival of cells which have already switched. It appears that isotype switch recombination (to any downstream isotype) involves a common switch recombinase (51) which is induced by LPS, and that IL-4 somehow 'opens up' the S regions of the $C_{\gamma 1}$

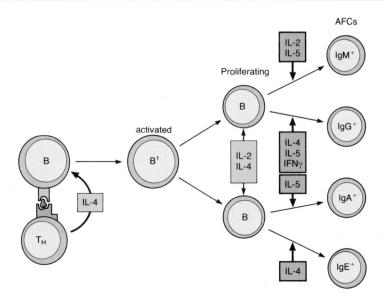

Figure 3.7.   A (speculative) scheme of current understanding of the role of cytokines in the control of various aspects of the primary B cell response to antigen. A resting B cell receives (undefined) activating signals during cognate T cell – B cell interaction, one of which may be IL-4. The various stages of the subsequent proliferation and differentiation of the clonal progeny of this cell are controlled by the cytokines shown in boxes, often acting in synergy, or antagonizing each other, to ultimately produce AFC secreting the different isotypes shown on the right.

and C_ϵ genes. The mechanisms involved in the actions of IL-5 and IFN_γ have not been established.

These results therefore strongly suggest that isotype regulation *in vivo* is controlled by a balance of various lymphokines secreted by T_{H1} and T_{H2} cells. This is supported by evidence for the importance of IFN_γ in IgG2a production and of IL-4 in IgE responses *in vivo* (31).

4.6 Role of cytokines in antibody responses: a synthesis

At present it thus appears that a multiplicity of cytokines modulate the responses of B cells to antigen. Much more work clearly needs to be done before any coherent picture emerges of how this cytokine network operates *in vivo*. The validity of any attempt to produce an overall synthesis of this field at present (*Figure 3.7*) must therefore be treated with considerable suspicion. Nevertheless, certain facts have emerged which will probably stand the test of time. These may be summarized as follows:

1. IL-4 is currently the best candidate for a molecule which acts early in the stimulation of resting B cells, and synergizes with antigen to induce their activation. It also somehow 'imprints' its later effects on isotype switching at an early stage of the activation cascade.
2. IL-5, IL-6, IL-2, and IFN_γ are clearly molecules which exert their multiple

Table 3.4. Characteristics of TI and TD antigens

Characteristic	TI-1 Ag	TI-2 Ag	TD Ag
Repeating epitopes	yes	yes	generally no
B cell mitogen	yes/no	no	no
Poorly degradable	yes/no	yes	no
Ab response	IgM + + +	IgM + + +	IgM + +
	IgG ±	IgG ±	IgG + +
Elicit memory	no	no	yes
Examples	DNP-LPS	DNP-Ficoll	SRBC
	Brucella abortus	dextrans	DNP-BSA
		levan	HGG

effects on pre-activated B cells, but how they do this is unclear. The concept of a lymphokine cascade, with one cytokine inducing responsiveness to later acting ones, is certainly an attractive one for which there is some evidence (38). Synergistic effects (e.g. between IL-4 and IL-5) or antagonistic effects (e.g. between IL-4 and IFN$_\gamma$) are probably also important.

3. T_H cell subsets are important in fine-tuning B cell responses, presumably as a result of the spectrum of lymphokines they secrete. The factors which control the emergence of T_{H1} or T_{H2} cells *in vivo* are not well understood. Nevertheless, the function of these subsets must be to programme the production of appropriate responses according to the nature of the antigen, its route of entry into the body, and its persistence. Thus, on the one hand, it is likely that parasite antigens favour the production of T_{H2} cells, with resultant IgE antibody formation and eosinophilia. On the other hand, T_{H1} cells are probably most important for anti-viral immunity, both as mediators of DTH responses and to elicit an appropriate antibody response (IgG2a in the mouse). Finally, the two T cell subsets undoubtedly control each others' activities: an example is the inhibition by IFN$_\gamma$ of the actions of IL-4.

5. TI antibody responses

The concept of TI-1 and TI-2 antigens was introduced in Chapter 2. TI antigens are generally polymeric bacterial products: some TI-1 antigens are polyclonal B cell activators at high concentrations (e.g. LPS), whilst TI-2 antigens (e.g. dextrans, pneumococcal capsular polysaccharides) are not (*Table 3.4*). In addition, TI-2 antigens persist for long periods in the body because they are not degraded in macrophages. The capacity of these antigens to stimulate antibody responses in the relative absence of T cells (e.g. in athymic mice) is undoubtedly a reflection of their polymeric nature: the presence of repeating epitopes therefore enables TI antigens to cause substantial cross-linking of sIg receptors, rather like anti-Ig antibodies (see Section 2.3). However, there is evidence that responses to TI antigens may also be modulated by T cell-derived cytokines. The cross-linking capacity of TI-2 antigens is also relevant to their potency in

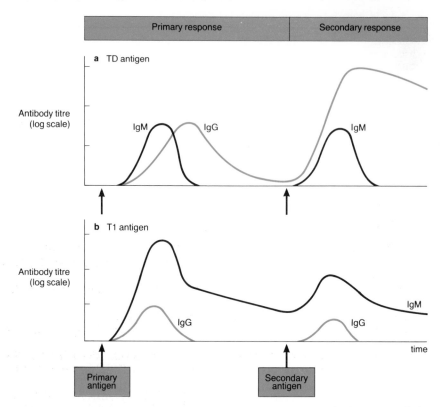

Figure 3.8.   Characteristics of TD and TI antibody responses in the mouse. Primary immunization with a TD antigen (panel **a**) induces relatively short-lived IgM and IgG antibody responses. Secondary immunization induces a larger, higher affinity, predominantly IgG antibody response, resulting from re-stimulation of B memory cells (see Chapter 4). TI antigens, in contrast, generally elicit long-lived primary IgM responses, poor IgG responses, and they do not induce classical memory (panel **b**).

inducing antigen-specific B cell unresponsiveness, even in mature B cells (see Chapter 5). The induction of specific anti-DNP antibody responses to TI-1 antigens such as DNP-LPS additionally involves the concentration (focusing) of the mitogenic activities of LPS by sIg receptors of hapten-specific B cells.

TI antigens elicit predominantly IgM antibody responses, which are often long-lived (*Figure 3.8*). In line with the known functions of T cells in isotype switching, the minimal IgG responses elicited by TI antigens consist largely of immediately downstream isotypes, such as IgG3 (52), as occurs in B cells polyclonally stimulated with LPS. Furthermore, TI antigens generally fail to establish immunological memory (Chapter 4).

TI-2 antigens localize selectively in macrophages in the marginal zone of the spleen (53; Chapter 4). Antibody responses to these antigens are produced predominantly by a sIgM⁺sIgD⁻ sessile population of B cells in the marginal zones of this organ (54). B cells responsive to TI-2 antigens emerge relatively late in ontogeny in both mouse and man. This is probably clinically relevant to the predisposition of newborn infants to infections of encapsulated bacteria.

6. Further reading

Vitetta,E.S., Fernandez-Botran,R., Myers,C.D. and Sanders,V.M. (1989) *Adv. Immunol.*, **45**, 1.
Moller,G. (ed.) (1987) *Immunol. Rev.*, **99**.
Mosmann,T.R. and Coffman,R.L. (1989) *Ann. Rev. Immunol.*, **7**, 145.

7. References

1. Gordon,J. and Guy,G.R. (1987) *Immunol. Today*, **8**, 339.
2. Subbarao,B. and Mosier,D.E. (1982) *Immunol. Rev.*, **69**, 81.
3. DeFranco,A.L., Kung,J.T. and Paul,W.E. (1982) *Immunol. Rev.*, **64**, 161.
4. Brunswick,M., Finkelman,F.D., Highest,P.F., Inman,J.K. and Dintzis,H.M. (1988) *J. Immunol.*, **140**, 3364.
5. Klaus,G.G.B., Bijsterbosch,M.K., O'Garra,A., Harnett,M.M. and Rigley,K.P. (1987) *Immunol. Rev.*, **99**, 19.
6. Harnett,M.M. and Klaus,G.G.B. (1988) *J. Immunol.*, **140**, 3135.
7. Klaus,G.G.B., O'Garra,A., Bijsterbosch,M.K. and Holman,M. (1986) *Eur. J. Immunol.*, **16**, 92.
8. Bijsterbosch,M.K., Meade,C.J., Turner,G.A. and Klaus,G.G.B. (1985) *Cell*, **41**, 999.
9. Klemsz,M.J., Justement,L.B., Palmer,E. and Cambier,J.C. (1989) *J. Immunol.*, **143**, 1032.
10. Gudat,F.G., Harris,T.N., Harris,S. and Hummeler,K. (1970) *J. Exp. Med.*, **132**, 448.
11. Early,P., Rogers,J., Davis,M., Calame,K. and Bond,M. (1980) *Cell*, **20**, 313.
12. Wall,R., Choi,E., Carter,C., Kuehl,M. and Rogers,J. (1980) *Cold Spring Harbor Symp. Quant. Biol.*, **45**, 879.
13. Benner,R., Coutinho,A., Rijnbeek,A.M., Van Oudenaren,A. and Hooijkas,H. (1981) *Eur. J. Immunol.*, **11**, 799.
14. Coutinho,A. and Forni,L. (1982) *EMBO J.*, **1**, 1251.
15. Zauderer,M. and Askonas,B.A. (1976) *Nature*, **260**, 611.
16. Honjo,T. and Kataoka,T. (1978) *Proc. Nat. Acad. Sci. USA*, **75**, 2140.
17. Claman,H.N., Chaperon,E.A. and Triplett,R.F. (1966) *Proc. Soc. Exp. Biol. Med.*, **122**, 2167.
18. Mitchison,N.A. (1971) *Eur. J. Immunol.*, **1**, 18.
19. Raff,M.C., Nase,S. and Mitchison,N.A. (1971) *Nature*, **230**, 50.
20. Mosier,D.E. and Coppelson,L.W. (1968) *Proc. Nat. Acad. Sci. USA*, **61**, 542.
21. Bjorkman,P.J., Saper,M.A., Samraoui,B., Bennett,W.S., Strominger,J.L. and Wiley,D.C. (1987) *Nature*, **329**, 506.
22. Kindred,B. and Schreffler,D.C. (1972) *J. Immunol.*, **109**, 940.
23. Sprent,J. (1978) *J. Exp. Med.*, **147**, 1142.
24. Chesnut,R.W. and Grey,H.M. (1981) *J. Immunol.*, **126**, 1075.
25. Lanzavecchia,A. (1985) *Nature*, **314**, 537.
26. Janeway,C.A., Murgita,R.A., Weinbaum,F., Asofsky,R. and Wigzell,H. (1977) *Proc. Nat. Acad. Sci. USA*, **74**, 4582.
27. Marrack,P., Skidmore,B. and Kappler,J.W. (1983) *J. Immunol.*, **130**, 2088.
28. Sanders,V.M., Snyder,J.M., Uhr,J.W. and Vitetta,E.S. (1986) *J. Immunol.*, **137**, 2395.

29. Kupfer,A., Swain,S.L., Janeway,C.A. and Singer,S.J. (1986) *Proc. Nat. Acad. Sci. USA,* **83**, 6080.
30. Cambier,J.C., Monroe,J.G. and Neale,M.J. (1982) *J. Exp. Med.,* **156**, 1635.
31. Niederhuber,J.E., Frelinger,J.A., Dugan,E., Coutinho,A. and Schreffler,D.C. (1975) *J. Immunol.,* **115**, 1672.
32. Cambier,J.C. and Lehmann,K.R. (1989) *J. Exp. Med.,* **170**, 873.
33. Cambier,J.C., Newell,M.K., Justement,L.B., McGuire,J.C., Leach,K.L. and Chen,Z.Z. (1987) *Nature,* **327**, 629.
34. O'Garra,A., Umland,S., DeFrance,T. and Christiansen,J. (1988) *Immunol. Today,* **9**, 45.
35. Howard,M., Farrar,W.L., Hilfiker,M., Johnson,B., Takatsu,K., Hamaoka,T. and Paul,W.E. (1982) *J. Exp. Med.,* **155**, 914.
36. Vitetta,E.S., Ohara,J., Myers,C.D., Layton,J.E., Krammer,P.H. and Paul,W.E. (1985) *J. Exp. Med.,* **162**, 1726.
37. Coffman,R.L. and Carty,J. (1986) *J. Immunol.,* **136**, 949.
38. Finkelman,F.D., Katona,I.M., Urban,J.F., Snapper,C.M., Ohara,J. and Paul,W.E. (1986) *Proc. Nat. Acad. Sci. USA,* **83**, 9675.
39. Paul,W.E. and Ohara,J. (1987) *Ann. Rev. Immunol.,* **5**, 429.
40. Swain,S.L., McKenzie,D.J., Dutton,R.W., Tonkonogy,S.L. and English,M. (1988) *Immunol. Rev.,* **102**, 77.
41. Murray,P.D., McKenzie,D.T., Swain,S.L. and Kagnoff,M.F. (1987) *J. Immunol.,* **139**, 2669.
42. Sanderson,C.J., Campbell,H.D. and Young,I.G. (1988) *Immunol. Rev.,* **102**, 29.
43. Sanderson,C.J., O'Garra,A., Warren,D.J. and Klaus,G.G.B. (1986) *Proc. Nat. Acad. Sci. USA,* **83**, 437.
44. Kishimoto,T. and Hirano,T. (1988) *BioEssays,* **9**, 11.
45. Osawa,H. and Diamantstein,T. (1984) *J. Immunol.,* **132**, 2445.
46. Lowenthal,J.W., Zubler,R.H., Nabholz,M. and MacDonald,R.H. (1985) *Nature,* **315**, 669.
47. Loughnan,M.S. and Nossal,G.J.V. (1989) *Nature,* **340**, 76.
48. Stevens,T.L., Bossie,A., Sanders,V.M., Fernandez-Botran,R., Coffman,R.L., Mosmann,T.R. and Vitetta,E.S. (1988) *Nature,* **334**, 255.
49. Rabin,E.M., Mond,J.J., Ohara,J. and Paul,W.E. (1986) *J. Immunol.,* **137**, 1573.
50. Mosmann,T.R. and Coffman,R.L. (1987) *Immunol. Today,* **8**, 223.
51. Shimizu,A. and Honjo,T. (1984) *Cell,* **36**, 801.
52. Mongini,P.K.A., Paul,W.E. and Metcalf,E.S. (1982) *J. Exp. Med.,* **155**, 884.
53. Humphrey,J.H. and Grennan,D. (1981) *Eur. J. Immunol.,* **11**, 221.
54. Lane,P.J.L., Gray,D., Oldfield,S. and MacLennan,I.C.M. (1986) *Eur. J. Immunol.,* **16**, 1569.

4

Memory and regulation of antibody responses

1. Introduction

Immunological memory refers to the capacity of a primarily immunized individual to give an accelerated, enhanced, and more efficient (secondary or anamnestic) immune response following re-exposure to the antigen (see *Figure 3.8*). The establishment of memory is therefore crucial to successful vaccination strategies. Memory is due to

(1) clonal expansion of antigen-responsive primary T and/or B cells following initial immunization;

(2) their concomitant differentiation into memory (or secondary) cells.

Memory cells are functionally (and hence phenotypically) different from primary lymphocytes, and from effector cells which mediate primary immune responses. In other words, the generation of memory cells occurs via a different antigen-driven differentiation pathway from that involved in the production of effector cells. The evidence for this last statement is clearer in the case of B cells than in the case of T cells, although there is growing evidence for the existence of phenotypically distinct T memory cells as well.

1.1 Hapten-carrier systems for studying B cell memory

The elicitation of sizeable primary antibody responses to most proteins requires relatively large doses of antigen (typically 100–200 µg in the mouse), given as a depot (e.g. as an alum precipitate) and the concomitant administration of an adjuvant (such as *Bordetella pertussis*). This elicits IgM and modest levels of low-affinity IgG antibodies (see Chapter 3, Section 5). Mice immunized in this fashion with hapten – protein conjugates have been widely used to study memory induction. After 1 – 6 months lymphocytes from these animals are injected into irradiated syngeneic animals, together with a low dose (1 – 10 µg) of antigen in saline. This experimental approach has established the following points.

1. The elicitation of optimal secondary antibody responses requires that both the hapten-specific B cells and carrier-specific T_H cells are from immunized, MHC-compatible individuals (see Chapter 3).
2. The recipient animals must be challenged with the hapten coupled to the same carrier used for T_H cell priming (linked recognition, see Chapter 3).
3. The antibodies made by the transferred B cells are mostly IgG and have much higher affinities for the hapten than antibodies produced during a primary response.

2. Properties of memory B cells

Primary B cells are relatively sessile and many are short-lived (see Chapter 2), whilst secondary B cells enter the re-circulating pool of lymphocytes and are longer-lived (1). In consequence, thoracic duct lymph is a rich source of memory B cells. The long duration of memory therefore reflects the existence of long-lived B cells (and T cells). However, it is not entirely clear to what extent the persistence of memory is dependent on periodical re-stimulation with antigen, either exogenously, or from depots within the lymphoid tissues (see below).

The induction of secondary B cells is T cell-dependent. Thus, athymic (*nu/nu*) mice not only fail to mount normal primary antibody responses to TD antigens, but do not generate memory cells to such antigens (2). The generation of secondary B cells can also be abrogated by treating mice with cobra venom factor (3) early during the priming period, which depletes them of the pivotal C3 component of the complement system (see below).

Like the activation of primary B cells, the re-activation of secondary B cells by antigen is also T cell-dependent and MHC-restricted. However, secondary B cells respond effectively to much lower concentrations of antigen than primary B cells, even in the absence of adjuvants. This is largely due to the higher *affinity* of sIg receptors on memory cells for antigen (Section 4), but may also reflect a greater density of sIg receptors on these cells. In any event, secondary B cells behave functionally as if they have a higher overall *avidity* for antigen than primary B cells (4). This is clearly important in order to enable memory cells to bind low concentrations of antigen in the presence of circulating antibodies which, being largely divalent, bind antigen less avidly than B cells carrying $c.$ 10^5 sIg receptors.

Secondary B cells are typically pre-committed to produce other isotypes apart from IgM, in particular IgG in the spleen and lymph nodes, and IgA in gut-associated tissues such as Peyers' patches. Cells committed to produce IgG of a particular subclass are believed to express sIg of that same subclass. Class switching at the level of sIg during memory cell induction probably does not involve switch recombination (see Chapter 3, Section 3.3.2), since secondary B cells can express multiple isotypes of sIg. Finally, memory B cells produce

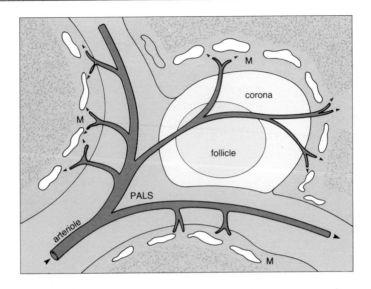

Figure 4.1. Structure of the white pulp of the spleen, showing vascular pathways. The white pulp is divided into periarteriolar lymphoid sheaths (PALS) whch consist of T cells and interdigitating (dendritic) cells, and follicles composed of B cells and FDC. After immunization germinal centres develop in the follicle centre, which is surrounded by a corona. Cells enter the spleen through the arterioles and initially penetrate the marginal zone (M) which surrounds both the PALS and the follicles. S = sinus of red pulp. (Modified from Van Rooijen *et al.*, 1989.)

higher-affinity antibodies than primary B cells. The significance of this finding is discussed in Section 4.

It will be evident that the definition of secondary B cells relies heavily on the functional properties of these cells and of their secreted products. Many laboratories have attempted to raise monoclonal antibodies which would distinguish primary from secondary B cells, without a great deal of success. This has hampered detailed characterization of memory cells.

3. Sites of secondary B cell generation in vivo

A second major problem in the elucidation of the pathway leading to the generation of secondary B cells is the lack of suitable *in vitro* models. This is because *in vivo* B cells develop into AFC or memory cells within different micro-environments in secondary lymphoid organs, and these are undoubtedly difficult to mimic in tissue culture.

The two major compartments of lymphocytes are broadly segregated in secondary lymphoid organs into T cell and B cell areas (*Figure 4.1*). Within the white pulp of the spleen the T cells are densely packed in the periarteriolar lymphoid sheaths, interspersed with interdigitating (dendritic) cells. Most B cells are organized into follicles. In an unimmunized individual the follicles are

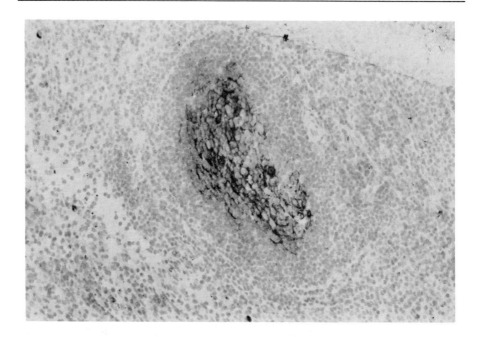

Figure 4.2.   Trapping of Ag – Ab complexes on FDC. Frozen section of rabbit spleen taken 7 days after immunization with human serum albumin (HSA), stained with HSA horseradish peroxidase, demonstrating typical dendritic localization of HSA – anti-HSA immune complexes on FDC within a germinal centre. (Taken from Van Rooijen *et al.*, 1989; with permission.)

composed of dense aggregates of resting B cells (primary follicles). After immunization, focal areas of activated, proliferating B cells appear within the (secondary) follicles and these are called *germinal centres* (reviewed in 5). These are sites of secondary B cell proliferation and differentiation (see below).

3.1 Follicular dendritic cells

Within the areas where germinal centres develop are unique, large, non-phagocytic cells, with ramifying, extensive processes, which are in intimate contact with surrounding B cells. These are follicular dendritic cells (FDC). FDC are phenotypically different from other dendritic cells (e.g. those in the T cell areas), or cells of the mononuclear phagocyte lineage. They carry distinct markers recognized by McAb, and also high levels of $Fc\gamma R$, and CR1, and CR2, but they are apparently not of bone marrow origin, unlike other dendritic cells (6).

FDC have the singular property of trapping and retaining undegraded antigens on their extensive cellular processes (*Figure 4.2*). They are the only cells in lymphoid tissues which can retain a depot of antigen for weeks and even months (reviewed in 7). They trap antigen in the form of antigen – antibody (Ag – Ab) complexes; this is complement-dependent, involving the pivotal C3 component (8). It is therefore likely that FDC bind Ag – Ab, or Ag – Ab – C3 complexes, via Fc and/or C3 receptors.

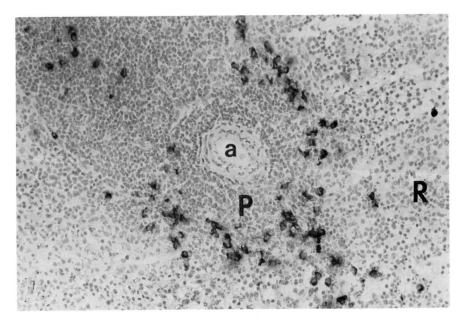

Figure 4.3. Localization of specific AFC in the periarteriolar lymphoid sheath of the spleen. Frozen section of a spleen from a rabbit immunized 6 days previously with human serum albumin, stained with HSA coupled to horseradish peroxidase. **a** = central arteriole, **P** = PALS, **R** = red pulp. (Taken from Van Rooijen *et al.*, 1989; with permission.)

3.2 Role of germinal centres in B cell memory

The functional significance of germinal centres puzzled immunologists for many years. Germinal centres are not sites of antibody formation, at least during the early stages of the response. Rather, in the spleen most AFC develop in the outer periarteriolar sheaths, and in the lymphoid sheaths surrounding the terminal arterioles (*Figure 4.3*; 9). Instead, it is now clear that germinal centres represent sites of B-memory-cell proliferation and differentiation.

Mice decomplemented by treatment with cobra venom factor do not trap Ag–Ab complexes on their FDC, and also fail to develop secondary B cells when immunized with a hapten–protein conjugate (reviewed in 10). Conversely, mice immunized with pre-formed Ag–Ab complexes localize these complexes on FDC very rapidly, and also develop secondary B cells more rapidly than animals immunized with antigen alone. There are therefore close correlations between C3-dependent uptake and retention of Ag–Ab complexes on FDC and the development of memory cells. Given the intimate physical association between FDC and follicular B cells, it seems likely that FDC present antigen to B lymphocytes, and that this provides one necessary signal for the development of germinal centres and the functional generation of memory cells.

3.3 Events leading to the development of B memory cells

The evidence summarized above suggests that the following sequence of events occurs following primary immunization (*Figure 4.4*; reviewed in 10,11).

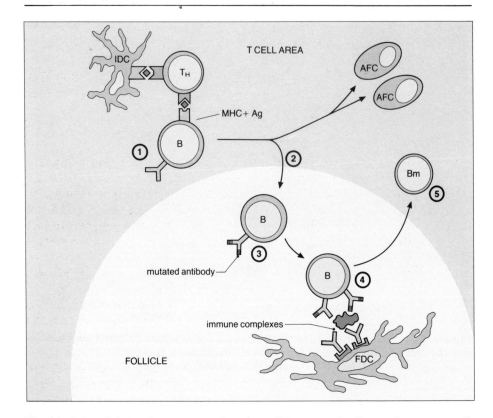

Figure 4.4. Schematic representation of possible events leading to B memory cell generation. (1) Primary B cells initially meet antigen in the T cell areas in spleen and lymph nodes: initial T cell activation may be via Ag presented on B cells or interdigitating cells (IDC, see Chapter 3). Some of the activated B cells mature into AFC, whilst others migrate into follicles (2). Here, in germinal centres, cells undergo somatic mutations (3) (Section 4.1), and high-affinity variants are selectively expanded by Ag – Ab complexes presented on FDC (4). Class switching (to IgG, and so on) occurs in germinal centres, and fully differentiated Bm cells leave the follicle to enter the re-circulating pool (5).

1. Primary B cells interact with T_H cells in the T cell areas of spleen and lymph nodes (perhaps with the aid of dendritic cells as additional APC) and some of these B cells develop into AFC (see Chapter 3). Other activated B cells migrate into follicles and undergo somatic mutations in their Ig V-region genes (Section 4.1).

2. If the antigen persists for long enough Ag – Ab complexes are formed. Provided these activate and bind C3 they are trapped on FDC in primary follicles. Transport of Ag – Ab complexes to FDC may itself be mediated by B cells.

3. FDC-associated antigen causes selective proliferation of high-affinity (mutated) B cells which migrate through the follicle, and promotes their differentiation along the memory cell pathway within germinal centres. Germinal centre blast cells shows all the characteristics of activated B cells: they are large

cells with high levels of MHC Class II antigens, low levels of sIgD, and some of them express sIgG (in spleen and lymph nodes) or sIgA (in gut lymphoid tissues) (12).

4. Germinal centre cells leave the follicles and enter the peripheral pool as long-lived memory cells. These cells remain in the resting state until they re-encounter antigen and are then reactivated to form AFC.

3.4 Micro-environmental factors controlling memory development

A crucial question therefore concerns the nature of the influences which determine whether B cells which encounter antigen outside follicles are stimulated to develop into AFC, whereas those which re-encounter antigen in follicles develop into secondary B cells. The composition of the antigen depot retained on FDC undoubtedly provides a key stimulus in the memory pathway. Since B cells are here confronted with antigen as an Ag–Ab–C3 complex, it is likely that interaction of the complex with CR1 and/or CR2 on B cells may modulate their activation. This is supported by evidence that monoclonal anti-CR1 or CR2 antibodies can polyclonally activate human B cells *in vitro*, and that complexed C3b or C3d act as growth and differentiation factors for pre-activated mouse B cells (reviewed in 13). The fact that EBV, which binds to CR2, polyclonally activates human B cells (see Chapter 3) is also in line with the importance of complement receptors in B cell activation.

Although germinal centres contain relatively few T cells, T cell signals are also crucial, since athymic mice cannot form memory cells or germinal centres in response to TD antigens. Also TI antigens (see Chapter 3, Section 5) do not induce true B cell memory. The nature of the T cell helper signals required for memory cell generation is totally unknown.

4. Affinity maturation during memory induction

Antibodies produced during the primary response generally exhibit a low affinity for antigen. The average affinity of the antibodies (in particular that of IgG) increases with time after priming, especially after a low dose of antigen. This process is called *affinity maturation* (reviewed in 14). For many years it was ascribed to the selective activation of high-affinity clonal precursors from the primary repertoire by decreasing concentrations of antigen. In other words, as antigen was catabolized and excreted, only those B cells with high-affinity sIg receptors would continue to be stimulated, and their antibodies would come to dominate later phases of the response.

4.1 The role of somatic mutations

More recently, the application of molecular biological analyses of antibody repertoire expression had led to a much clearer understanding of affinity maturation. The approach used to study this problem is to make hybridomas

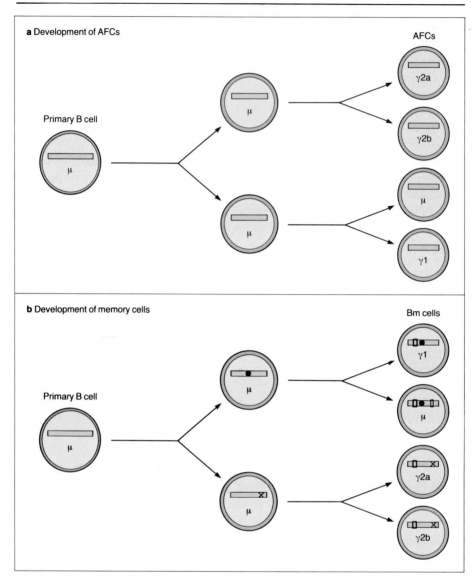

Figure 4.5.   Schematic representation of events occurring during clonal expansion of a primary B cell clone to form AFC (panel **a**) or memory cells (panel **b**). The bars depict a V-region gene, with individual somatic mutations shown as circles, squares, and so on. The Greek symbols depict the isotype of Ig produced by that cell. During the primary response intraclonal isotype switching from IgM to downstream isotypes occurs, but somatic mutations are rare. During memory cell formation individual clonal progeny undergo stepwise mutations, which may or may not be accompanied by class switching (modified from Rajewsky *et al.* (1987) *Science,* **238**, 1088).

from mice immunized for varying periods with antigen and then to sequence the V-regions of the monoclonal antibodies (reviewed in 15,16). These studies have shown that most antibodies produced during the first week of the primary response carry unmutated, germline V-regions, and are of relatively low affinity, as predicted. In contrast, high-affinity antibodies produced later in the primary response, and especially by secondary B cells invariably contain mutations in their V-regions. These somatic mutations show the following characteristics.

1. They occur at extremely high frequency (around 10^{-3} to 10^{-4} changes per base pair per cell division). This is two orders of magnitude higher than the frequency found in pre-B cells (17). Most are point mutations.

2. They are restricted to rearranged V-regions (both V_H and V_L), and their immediate 5′ and 3′ flanking sequences and are clustered in mutational 'hotspots'.

3. They occur in IgM antibodies, so that hypermutation is not necessarily associated with isotype switching, even though this may occur at the same time.

4. Mutations are introduced stepwise during clonal proliferation. Single base changes can alter the affinity of an antibody by a factor of 10-fold, and can even change the specificity of the antibody. Examples of somatic mutations and class switching during the activation of primary B cell clones to form AFC or secondary B cells are depicted in *Figure 4.5*.

It is therefore now clear that the induction of this localized hypermutation mechanism is a key process during the establishment of the secondary B cell repertoire, and that it explains affinity maturation. Indeed, we can now define a secondary B cell as one which has mutated its V-region genes. What appears to happen during the generation of B cell memory is that somatic mutants of primary B cell clones, expressing higher-affinity sIg receptors, are selectively expanded by falling levels of antigen. The antibody products of these cells thus dominate late primary and secondary antibody responses.

4.2 Does somatic mutation occur in germinal centres?

Circumstantial evidence strongly suggests that somatic mutations occur in germinal centres (11). There is a temporal correlation between the appearance of germinal centres and the onset of somatic mutations. Also, germinal centres represent the only sites where B cells proliferate at a rate consistent with the high mutation frequencies observed. Nothing is known about the stimuli (presumably T cell-derived) which initiate the hypermutation process. Nevertheless, the antigen depot on FDC must play a pivotal role in the process of affinity maturation. As further discussed below, rising levels of antibodies together with falling concentrations of antigen will combine to limit the effective concentration of epitopes available for B cell recognition. This will provide a key selective factor in promoting the expansion of high-affinity mutants.

5. Regulation of antibody responses

5.1 End-product feedback

All immune responses are tightly controlled. A major factor in the control of antibody responses is end-product feedback (18). In other words, antibodies

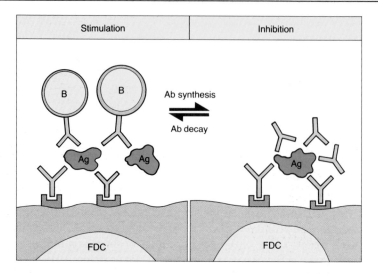

Figure 4.6. The dynamic role of FDC-bound antigen in long-term regulation of antibody production. As antibody production commences antigen is bound as Ag – Ab complexes to CR and/or FcR on FDC: free epitopes on these complexes are available for stimulating B cells (left). Rising antibody levels progressively mask epitopes on the Ag, thereby inhibiting B cell stimulation (right). Subsequently, as Ab levels fall epitopes on the Ag are again revealed (modified from 7).

themselves inhibit the further formation of antibodies. Broadly speaking, IgG antibodies are more effective in inducing feedback than IgM. This may be partly due to their higher affinity for antigen since high-affinity IgG antibodies are more suppressive than low-affinity ones.

5.1.1 Effects of antibodies on the fate of antigens

The mechanisms involved in antibody feedback are complex. Firstly, high concentrations of antibodies promote the uptake of antigen by mononuclear phagocytes (opsonization), thereby leading to their more rapid removal. Secondly, although antibodies promote the retention of antigens on FDC, ultimately they can mask epitopes on the trapped Ag – Ab complex. Hence, the antigen depots retained on FDC play a crucial role in long-term regulation of antibody production, in addition to their role in memory cell priming (7): for example, certain antigens, such as human gamma globulin, elicit cyclical antibody responses in experimental animals, where the primary response is followed by 'spontaneous' subsequent waves of antibody production (19). These cycles are due to the persistence of antigen on FDC. Rising levels of antibodies mask epitopes on the antigen and inhibit antibody formation. As antibody levels fall, epitopes are again exposed and the persisting antigen stimulates a further wave of antibody secretion (*Figure 4.6*).

5.1.2. Effects of antibodies on B cells

The third mechanism involved in antibody feedback is direct inhibition of B cell activation via an Fc-dependent mechanism. Pioneering studies by Sinclair *et al.*

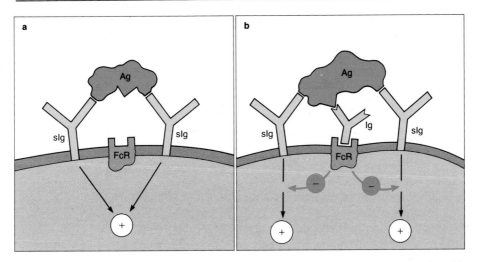

Figure 4.7. Schematic depiction of the control of B cell activation by Ag–Ab complexes. **a** As discussed in Chapter 3 cross-linking of sIg receptors by Ag, or F(ab')$_2$ anti-Ig, induces inositol phospholipid hydrolysis and B cell activation. **b** In contrast, Ag–Ab complexes containing IgG antibodies form a lattice, cross-linking both sIg and FcγR. This abrogates phosphoinositide breakdown and B cell activation. Note that only B cells carrying receptors specific for the Ag in the complex will be affected. Similar mechanisms may operate in the anti-Id-induced feedback of antibody production.

(20, reviewed in 21) showed that although high concentrations of F(ab')$_2$ fragments of antibodies can inhibit antibody responses by the mechanisms outlined above, feedback by low concentrations of IgG requires antibodies with an intact Fc region. This is because Ag–IgG antibody complexes cross-link both sIg and FcγR on B cells and this inhibits B cell activation (*Figure 4.7*). The mechanisms involved have been elucidated using intact (IgG) RaMIg, which binds to both sIg and FcR on murine B cells with high affinity (22). The co-cross-linking of the two types of receptors inhibits sIg-mediated phosphoinositide breakdown, subsequent second messenger production (see Chapter 3, Section 2.3), and B cell activation (23).

Such Fc-dependent regulation of B cell activation may also occur in germinal centres, although there is no direct evidence for this. It is noteworthy that Fc-dependent feedback can be counteracted by T cells or their products, most notably IL-4 (24). This suggests that the degree of B cell activation achieved under particular micro-environmental conditions may be determined by a balance of positive signals (emanating from sIg and T cell-derived cytokines) and negative ones (e.g. those emanating from the FcR).

5.2 Anti-idiotypic control of antibody production

Immunoglobulins themselves are highly immunogenic antigens. Antigenic determinants associated with the V-regions are called idiotypic determinants (or idiotopes) and are recognized by anti-idiotypic antibodies (anti-Id). A single anti-Id may recognize a unique clonal product (private idiotype) or a set of antibodies (public idiotype). Studies in mice, and similar observations in man, have shown that both T and B cells exist which can recognize self-idiotypes (reviewed in 25). Thus inbred mice can be immunized with their own McAb to generate anti-Id antibodies, and these in turn can be used to raise anti(anti)-idiotypic antibodies, and so on. This sort of observation led Jerne (26) to postulate that the immune system consists of a network of interacting idiotypes. His network theory envisaged that Id – anti-Id interactions could play central roles both in shaping the developing pre-immune repertoire (see Chapter 2, Section 6.3) and also in regulating induced immune responses in the adult. A detailed discussion of idiotype networks is outside the scope of this volume, so only a few key points will be considered here.

Much of the evidence for idiotypic regulation of antibody production has come from experimental systems in mice, using antigens which produce relatively homogeneous antibody responses, such as PC or dextran (reviewed in 27). Some 90% of anti-PC antibodies in Balb/c mice, for example, carry a single idiotype (T15). Giving anti-T15Id antibodies to adult mice causes temporary suppression of the anti-PC antibody response, whilst in neonatal mice it induces long-lasting suppression of the Id (28). In addition, there is evidence that anti-Id antibodies can be produced during the course of an anti-PC antibody response (29). Ag – Ab complexes can also induce anti-Id antibodies to the antibody, thus raising the possibility that the antigen depot on FDC may play a role in network control (30). In various systems anti-Id antibodies have been found to cause either enhancement or suppression, depending on rather poorly understood variables (27). Finally, naturally occurring anti-Id antibodies have been found in human sera, in particular in a variety of autoimmune diseases, such as rheumatoid arthritis.

It is thus clear that the immune system (especially during early life) has the capacity to respond to self-idiotypes. It is therefore still conceptually attractive to postulate that anti-Id antibodies and/or T cells may serve as immunoregulatory forces to shape and control antibody responses. However, there is still little definitive evidence that auto-anti-idiotypic immune responses occur during responses to typical environmental antigens, or indeed act as important means of immunoregulation. One major problem is that common protein antigens induce heterogeneous antibody responses, thereby diminishing the likelihood that individual idiotypes would reach a threshold of immunogenicity during the course of the immune response.

5.3 Immunoregulation by T cells

Most phases of antigen-dependent B cell stimulation are controlled by T cells, as has been discussed at some length. However, the precise role of T cells in long-term regulation of antibody responses is relatively poorly understood. There is currently growing evidence for the concept that the division of T_H cells into T_{H1} and T_{H2} subsets plays a major role in fine-tuning B cell responses (reviewed in 31). The secretion of different isotypes of antibodies following primary B cell activation *in vitro* can be markedly affected by various lymphokines secreted by the two subsets of T_H cells (see Chapter 3). This is further supported by evidence for the importance of IFNγ in IgG2a production and of IL-4 in IgE responses *in vivo*. In addition, the two subsets of T cells can cross-regulate each others' activities (31). This raises the attractive possibility that control of antibody production can be mediated by cross-talk between different types of T helper cells, acting in concert with the antibody feedback mechanisms outlined above.

Finally, T-suppressor cells should be mentioned, at least for completeness. The concept of a distinct population of T cells which suppress immune responses is conceptually attractive but finds relatively little support in contemporary dogma. The interested reader is referred to two recent reviews which discuss the problem (32,33).

6. Further reading

Kosco,M.H. and Tew,J.G. (1989) *Ann. Rev. Immunol.,* **7**, 91.
Van Rooijen,N., Claasen,E., Kraal,G. and Dijkstra,C.D. (1989) *Prog. Histochem. Cytochem.,* **19** (3).

7. References

1. Strober,S. (1975) *Transplant. Rev.,* **24**, 84.
2. Thorbecke,G.J. and Lerman,S.P. (1976) *Adv. Exp. Biol.,* **73A**, 83.
3. Klaus,G.G.B. and Humphrey,J.H. (1977) *Immunology,* **33**, 31.
4. Klinman,N.R. (1972) *J. Exp. Med.,* **136**, 241.
5. Nieuwenhuis,P. and Opstelten,D. (1984) *Amer. J. Anat.,* **170**, 421.
6. Humphrey,J.H. and Sundaram,V. (1985) *Adv. Exp. Med. Biol.,* **186**, 167.
7. Tew,J.G., Phipps,R.P. and Mandel,T.E. (1980) *Immunol. Rev.,* **53**, 175.
8. Papamichail,M., Gutierrez,C., Embling,P., Johnson,P. and Holborow,E.J. (1975) *Scand. J. Immunol.,* **4**, 343.
9. Van Rooijen,N., Claasen,E. and P.Eikelenboom,P. (1986) *Immunol. Today,* **7**, 193.
10. Klaus,G.G.B., Humphrey,J.H., Kunkl,A. and Dongworth,D.W. (1980) *Immunol. Rev.,* **53**, 3.
11. MacLennan,I.C.M. and Gray,D. (1986) *Immunol. Rev.,* **91**, 61.
12. Kraal,G., Weissman,I.L. and Butcher,E.C. (1982) *Nature,* **298**, 377.
13. Klaus,G.G.B. and Humphrey,J.H. (1986) *Immunol. Today,* **7**, 163.
14. Siskind,G.D. and Benacerraf,B. (1969) *Adv. Immunol.,* **10**, 1.
15. Berek,C. and Milstein,C. (1987) *Immunol. Rev.,* **96**, 24.
16. Allen,D., Cumano,A., Dildrop,R., Kocks,C., Rajewsky,K., Rajewsky,N., Roes,J., Sablitsky,F. and Siekevitz,M. (1987) *Immunol. Rev.,* **96**, 5.
17. Wabl,M., Burrows,P.D., von Gabain,A. and Steinberg,C. (1985) *Proc. Nat. Acad. Sci. USA,* **82**, 479.
18. Uhr,J.W. and Moller,G. (1968) *Adv. Immunol.,* **8**, 81.
19. Romball,C.G. and Weigle,W.O. (1973) *J. Exp. Med.,* **138**, 1426.
20. Sinclair,N.R.StC. and Chan,P.L. (1971) *Adv. Exp. Biol. Med. Sci.,* **12**, 609.
21. Sinclair,N.R.StC. and Panaskoltsis,A. (1987) *Immunol. Today,* **8**, 76.
22. Phillips,N.E. and Parker,D.C. (1984) *J. Immunol.,* **132**, 627.
23. Bijsterbosch,M.K. and Klaus,G.G.B. (1985) *J. Exp. Med.,* **162**, 1825.
24. O'Garra,A., Rigley,K.P., Holman,M., McLaughlin,J. and Klaus,G.G.B. (1987) *Proc. Nat. Acad. Sci. USA,* **84**, 6254.
25. Bona,C. (1981) *Idiotypes and Lymphocytes.* Academic Press, New York.

26. Jerne,N.K. (1974) *Ann. Immunol. (Inst. Pasteur),* **125C**, 373.
27. Rajewsky,K. and Takemori,T. (1983) *Ann. Rev. Immunol.,* **1**, 569.
28. Augustin,A. and Cosenza,H. (1976) *Eur. J. Immunol.,* **6**, 497.
29. Kelsoe,G. and Cerny,J. (1979) *Nature,* **279**, 333.
30. Klaus,G.G.B. (1978) *Nature,* **272**, 265.
31. Mosmann,T.R. and Coffman,R.L. (1989) *Ann. Rev. Immunol.,* **7**, 145.
32. Green,D.R., Flood,P.M. and Gershon,R.K. (1983) *Ann. Rev. Immunol.,* **1**, 439.
33. Batchelor,J.R., Lombardi,G. and Lechler,R.I. (1989) *Immunol. Today,* **10**, 37.

5

B cell tolerance

1. Introduction

A cardinal feature of the immune system is its capacity to respond to foreign antigens, whilst not responding to self-components (self – non-self discrimination). Non-responsiveness to self-antigens (self-tolerance) is principally established by the deletion and/or silencing of clones of autoreactive lymphocytes before they become immunocompetent.

Immunological tolerance is therefore the opposite of immune responsiveness: in operational terms tolerance refers to the induction of a state of specific unresponsiveness (at the level of either cell-mediated and/or humoral immunity) by exposure to an antigen, which can be a self-antigen or, experimentally, a foreign antigen. The induction of tolerance therefore follows the same rules of antigenic (or epitopic) specificity as the elicitation of immunity. Furthermore, as one might predict, antigens can make either T and/or B cells unresponsive.

2. T cell versus B cell tolerance

The classical explanation for self-tolerance was formulated as part of the clonal selection theory by Burnett and Fenner (1). Phrased in contemporary terms, as the primary pre-immune V-region repertoire is generated during (T or B) lymphocyte ontogeny, those clones with receptors of sufficiently high affinity for self-antigens are somehow silenced. Lederberg (2) first postulated that the purging of autoreactive clones occurs during a tolerance-sensitive period in the life of the developing lymphocytes. Only cells that pass through this window of tolerance susceptibility become immunocompetent and enter the peripheral pool.

The commonest experimental approach used to study tolerance is to give animals a tolerogenic form of an antigen (the 'tolerogen') followed by subsequent challenge with an immunogenic form of the antigen. Good examples of tolerogens are foreign Ig, such as human gamma globulin (HGG), which can be used to study tolerance to the protein itself, or to haptenic groups attached to it. If HGG is freed of aggregated protein by ultracentrifugation it is a powerful tolerogen which can induce both T and B cell tolerance in adult mice (3). Heat-aggregated HGG (or HGG given with an adjuvant), on the other hand, is a potent immunogen.

Tolerance to many self-antigens in T cells is clearly established during their differentiation in the thymus. Here subtle and still poorly understood selection procedures occur: these spare the clones of cells which can recognize foreign peptides associated with self-MHC antigens, and functionally eliminate those clones which react with self-antigens. Self-reactive clones die in the thymus, probably via a process of programmed cell death caused by DNA fragmentation (apoptosis).

The question of T cell tolerance is a large and complex one which cannot be discussed in greater detail here (reviewed in 4). However, it obviously cannot be completely divorced from B cell tolerance since with many (TD) antigens functional silencing of T_H cells is sufficient to effectively render the B cell compartment unresponsive. Indeed, studies with antigens such as HGG have shown that much lower doses of antigen are required to induce T cell tolerance than to inactivate B cells (5). This fundamental observation implies that the antigen dose threshold for inducing unresponsiveness in T cells to self-antigens may also be lower than that for B cells. In consequence, for many self-antigens tolerance may be maintained solely or largely at the level of T cells.

2.1 Do B cells become tolerant to self-antigens?

Self-tolerance is not absolute: the fact that both man and animals suffer from a variety of autoimmune diseases tells us that the immune system is not foolproof and that autoreactivity can and does occur. Normal individuals have B cells which bind autoantigens which are present in low concentrations, such as thyroglobulin and self-idiotypes, but lack B cells that bind abundant antigens such as serum albumen (6,7). In addition, hybridomas made with lymphocytes of unimmunized mice often bind to a variety of autoantigens, especially if the cells are from young animals. As has been discussed in Chapter 2, there is evidence that the repertoire of B cells early in ontogeny is skewed towards self-reactivity.

It is therefore tempting to argue that only abundant self-antigens achieve the necessary threshold to tolerize developing B cells. In addition, since tolerization of B cells requires cross-linking of sIg (see below), antigens which are effectively monomeric (such as small globular proteins) may not be tolerogenic. However, things are not so simple. A striking example of an authentic and abundant self-antigen which does not induce B cell tolerance is the C5 complement component. This is present in serum at concentrations of $50-85$ μg/ml in normal mice, whilst some strains lack C5. Such C5-deficient mice are not tolerant to the protein, whilst C5-sufficient animals are tolerant. However, the unresponsiveness is due to T cell and not B cell tolerance (8).

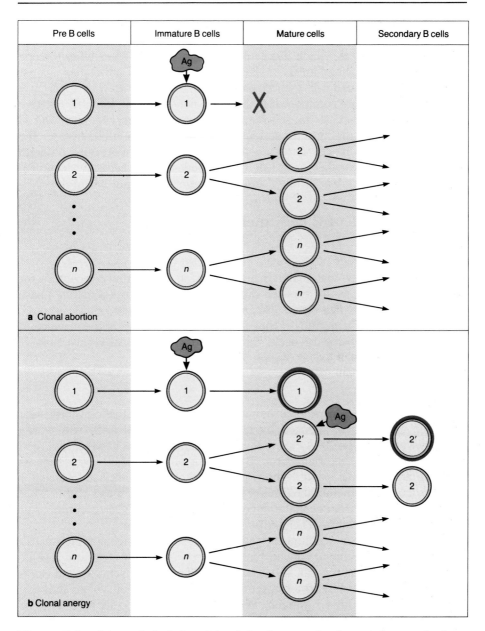

Figure 5.1. Schematic depiction of clonal abortion **a**, or clonal anergy **b** as mechanisms for B cell tolerance. In **a** an immature autoreactive B cell clone (1) which encounters self-antigen is killed soon after it expresses sIgM receptors. In **b** the self-antigen does not kill the cell, but renders it unresponsive to future encounter with antigen (ringed in red). This may also occur in immature B cells, or in mature cells, even after their initial encounter with antigen; for example, in a clone (2′) which has undergone somatic mutation(s).

The difficulty in interpreting currently available information concerning the extent of self-tolerance in B cells probably stems from the inbuilt degeneracy of the immune system, which has evolved a high degree of flexibility to cope with novel environmental antigens. Hence, the affinities of antibodies against a particular antigen can vary enormously and cross-reactivities with apparently unrelated antigens are common. It is therefore not surprising that self-reactive B cells exist. In fact, if all self-reactive clones were purged from the B cell compartment this would seriously compromise the diversity of the antibody repertoire. B cells with high-affinity receptors are more susceptible to tolerization than low-affinity cells (9). In consequence, most naturally occurring autoantibodies are of low affinity, and hence presumably not harmful.

3. Mechanisms of B cell tolerance

3.1 In immature B cells

It is therefore likely that many B cells carrying high-affinity receptors for abundant self-antigens are silenced during a critical tolerance-sensitive phase in their development. This occurs just as the cells have expressed sIgM receptors (see Chapter 2) and especially if they encounter the antigen in the absence of T cell help (10). Silencing can occur via two mechanisms—by *clonal abortion* (i.e. deletion) and by *clonal anergy* (*Figure 5.1*).

3.1.1 Clonal abortion

The most extreme experimental example of clonal abortion is the total abrogation of B cell development induced by treatment of neonatal mice with anti-μ antibodies (see Chapter 2). A clue to the possible mechanisms involved emerged from *in vitro* studies. Culturing mature B cells with anti-Ig for short periods causes patching and capping of sIg. These cells then clear the antibody – receptor complex from their membranes and re-express their sIg receptors within 24 h. In contrast, B cells from neonatal mice fail to re-express sIgM receptors after their modulation by anti-μ (11) and probably eventually die.

These results therefore suggest that high doses of antigens which cause substantial cross-linking of sIg can abort the development of immature B cells. There is evidence that this can also occur with self-antigens. Nemazee and Burki (12) generated mice carrying a transgene for the H and L chains of an antibody to the H-2^k MHC Class I antigen. Whilst 20 – 50% of B cells in H-2^d mice expressed the transgene, these cells could not be detected in (H-2^d × H-2^k) F1 transgenic mice. The interpretation of this experiment is that the relevant B cells were eliminated as a result of encountering the H-2^k 'neoself' antigen during their development in the marrow.

3.1.2 Clonal anergy

This refers to a poorly understood form of unresponsiveness where immature (or mature, see below) B cells exposed to tolerogen somehow store 'negative

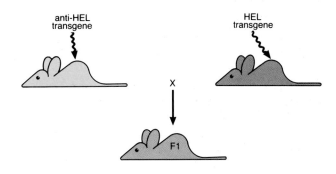

Anti-HEL B cells	Anti-HEL parental	F1
Number	+++	+++
Response to HEL	+++	−
sIg M	+++	±
sIg D	+++	+++

Figure 5.2.   The Goodnow *et al.* double transgenic experiment to demonstrate clonal anergy in B cells. One strain of mice was transgenic for the hen-egg lysozyme (HEL) gene, whilst the other carried transgenes for anti-HEL V-regions, together with Cμ and Cδ. Most of the B cells in the latter expressed anti-HEL sIgM and sIgD receptors. The F1 hybrid progeny of these two strains also had high numbers of anti-HEL B cells, but these were unresponsive to HEL, and showed markedly reduced levels of sIgM receptors for HEL (see 15).

signals' which render them unresponsive to antigen, but which do not lead to their immediate death. This has been extensively studied with antigens such as deaggregated HGG both *in vivo* and *in vitro*. Mice injected with haptenated-HGG, for example, have normal levels of hapten-binding B cells in their lymphoid organs, but these cells fail to produce antibodies when challenged with immunogenic forms of the hapten (reviewed in 13). The establishment of anergy is an active process, which requires RNA and protein synthesis (14), and there is evidence that 'tolerant' B cells cannot cap their sIg receptors normally. These cells are not totally refractory to stimulation, however, but become enlarged, express increased levels of Ia antigens (i.e. become abortively activated), but do not proliferate normally in response to antigen or differentiate into AFC (12).

   Clonal anergy has also been demonstrated in transgenic mice. Goodnow *et al.* (15) constructed one line carrying a transgene for the antigen hen egg lysozyme (HEL). The second line was transgenic for a high-affinity anti-HEL McAb and some 90% of the B cells in these animals expressed both sIgM and sIgD with specificity for HEL. The two strains were mated so that the F1 progeny expressed both HEL (as a neo-self-antigen) and anti-HEL (*Figure 5.2*). These animals still possessed large numbers of anti-HEL B cells. However, these B cells were profoundly anergic when challenged with HEL in the presence or absence of T cell help. These anergic B cells expressed 10–20-fold lower levels of sIgM receptors than those from the singly transgenic animals.

It is still uncertain what determines whether B cells become anergic, rather than being deleted by contact with tolerogen. Obvious possibilities are the nature and/or the concentration of the antigen. Furthermore, the biochemical mechanisms leading to anergy are unknown. As discussed in Chapter 3 sIg receptors on mature B cells are typical Ca^{2+}-mobilizing receptors, which utilize phosphoinositide breakdown to generate intracellular second messengers. There is little information available about the biochemical consequences of engaging sIg receptors on immature B cells. Low concentrations of anti-Ig antibodies inhibit the spontaneous growth of certain phenotypically immature murine B cell lymphomas. Such cell lines have therefore been used as models for studying antigen-mediated B cell tolerance (although the fact that these are tumour cells should not be forgotten). These studies have shown that the inhibitory signal induced by anti-Ig occurs during the G_1 phase of the cell cycle. The nature of the signal is not known, but it does not appear to involve an increase in intracellular Ca^{2+} resulting from sIg cross-linking (reviewed in 16).

The induction of B cell tolerance by hapten-HGG may involve co-cross-linking of sIg and FcR by the tolerogen, since haptenated F(ab')$_2$ fragments of HGG are less potent B cell tolerogens (17). This could then interrupt sIg receptor signalling in a similar fashion to that described for inhibition of B cell activation by Ag–Ab complexes (see Chapter 4, Section 5). However, other protein carriers which do not bind to FcR can also induce B cell tolerance, so it is unlikely to be the sole mechanism.

3.2 In mature B cells

Although immature lymphocytes do pass through a tolerance-sensitive window in their development, mature lymphocytes (and even memory cells) can also be tolerized, although this may require higher concentrations of antigen. In B cells it seems that similar mechanisms are operative in immature and mature cells. Thus, antigens such as DNP-HGG can induce clonal anergy in B cells from adult mice (reviewed in 13). Polysaccharide TI-2 antigens (such as DNP-pneumococcal polysaccharide) are also very effective tolerogens for mature B cells, presumably because of their capacity to cause massive cross-linking of sIg, and also because they are not recognized by T_H cells. Small doses of these antigens markedly suppress anti-DNP antibody production elicited by antigens such as DNP–protein conjugates, even in pre-immunized animals (18). There is evidence that this is due to irreversible sIg modulation (and hence effectively clonal deletion) as was described for anti-Ig in immature B cells above (19).

The fact that mature, immunocompetent lymphocytes remain susceptible to silencing by antigen reflects the existence of a failsafe mechanism within the immune system. This presumably evolved to inactivate clones of autoreactive cells which escape tolerization during their development, perhaps because the self-antigen in question is not expressed in the milieu where the cells develop.

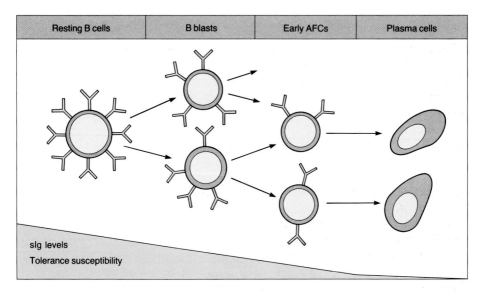

Resting B cells	B blasts	Early AFCs	Plasma cells

slg levels

Tolerance susceptibility

Figure 5.3.   Progressive loss of susceptibility of activated B cells to control by antigen. The unstimulated precursor cell is susceptible to tolerization (e.g. by high doses of a TI-2 antigen). Activated blasts progressively loses sIg (and hence the capacity to bind antigen) during successive rounds of division as they mature into plasma cells. Thus early AFC (which still express some sIg receptors) are susceptible to AFC blockade, whereas mature plasma cells are not.

In addition, in B cells the induction of somatic hypermutation in antibody V-region genes following antigen stimulation (Chapter 4) not only generates high-affinity variants, but also self-reactive, potentially pathogenic clones. Goodnow *et al.* (20) have used the HEL/anti-HEL transgenic mice discussed above to study tolerization of mature B cells. They found that transferring anti-HEL transgenic splenic B cells into HEL transgenic mice rapidly induced down-regulation of sIgM and clonal anergy. These results therefore dramatically confirm that immunocompetent B cells remain susceptible to tolerization by self-antigens.

3.3 Antibody-forming cell blockade

Classical tolerance normally results from the functional silencing of antigen-reactive precursor lymphocytes. However, B cells remain susceptible to control by antigen for some time after they have become activated, and even when they have started to secrete antibody at a high rate. This is because activated B cells continue to express sIg receptors during several rounds of division, albeit in decreasing levels, so that it is only the terminally differentiated plasma cells which lack sIg (*Figure 5.3*, 21).

   Experimentally, multi-valent antigens or Ag – Ab complexes can markedly decrease the amounts of antibodies secreted by AFC (22,23). This phenomenon (called AFC blockade) is particularly evident with TI-2 antigens, presumably because it requires extensive cross-linking of sIg receptors (Chapter 3, Section 5). The concentrations of antigen needed to induce AFC blockade are higher

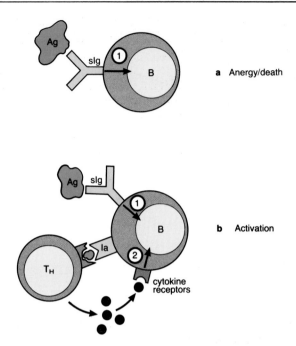

Figure 5.4. Contemporary version of the Bretscher – Cohn 'two signal' hypothesis determining the outcome of a lymphocyte's encounter with antigen. Shown is a B cell (mature or immature): binding of a critical level of Ag (signal 1) leads to anergy or death of that cell (**a**), unless it concurrently receives a second signal from an interacting T_H cell (**b**). A similar argument applies to T cells: binding of Ag alone induces anergy (or death?) unless the cell receives a second signal from an APC. This provides a potential failsafe mechanism to silence clones of autoreactive cells which have not been inactivated during the development of the primary repertoire (see 25).

than those needed to induce classical tolerance of precursor B cells. Blockade is not due to mopping up of secreted antibodies by cell-associated antigen, but rather reflects a decrease in the rate of antibody synthesis, which becomes irreversible with increasing time. The mechanisms are not known in detail. However, anti-Ig antibodies produce a similar effect (e.g. in B cells stimulated to secrete Ig by LPS) and this has been shown to be due to transcriptional regulation of mRNA for secreted IgM.

The importance of AFC blockade in immunoregulation is difficult to evaluate. It may represent another mechanism for fine-tuning antibody responses after their inception, and hence it may be part of a feedback loop (see Chapter 4, Section 5.1). It may also be important in responses to persistent antigens such as polysaccharides.

4. Concluding remarks

The immune system has evolved multiple strategies for controlling autoreactivity. Thus, some high-affinity autoreactive B cells are probably silenced during their differentiation in the marrow, where contact with self-antigen will induce deletion or anergy, depending on poorly understood factors. Mature B cells can also be inactivated, although this may require high concentrations of antigen. What is important in both cases is that B cells become unresponsive if they encounter antigen in the absence of a second signal, which is generally provided by a T_H cell, probably in the form of one or more cytokines (Chapter 3). This 'two signal' model of immune induction was first formulated by Bretscher and Cohn (24) and is illustrated in *Figure 5.4*. It explains why TI antigens are powerful B cell tolerogens (because they are not recognizd by T cells). It also predicts that if T cells are tolerant to a particular antigen, this in turn renders B cells specific for the antigen more susceptible to tolerization (for further discussion see 25).

5. Further reading

Nossal,G.J.V. (1983) *Ann. Rev. Immunol.*, **1**, 33.

6. References

1.   Burnett,F.M. and Fenner,F. (1949) *The Production of Antibodies.* (2nd edn.). Macmillan, Melbourne and London.
2.   Lederberg,J. (1959) *Science*, **129**, 1649.
3.   Dresser,D.W. (1962) *Immunology*, **5**, 161.
4.   Schwartz,R.H. (1989) *Cell*, **57**, 1073.
5.   Weigle,W.O. (1973) *Adv. Immunol.*, **16**, 61.
6.   Bankhurst,A.D., Torrigiani,G. and Allison,A.C. (1973) *Lancet*, **i**, 226.
7.   Roberts,I.M., Whittingham,S. and Mackay,I.R. (1973) *Lancet*, **ii**, 936.
8.   Harris,D.E., Cairns,L., Rosen,F.S. and Borel,Y. (1983) *J. Exp. Med.*
9.   Riley,R.L. and Klinman,N.R. (1986) *J. Immunol.*, **136**, 3147.
10. Metcalfe,E.S. and Klinman,N.R. (1976) *J. Exp. Med.*, **143**, 1327.
11. Sidman,C.L. and Unanue,E.R. (1975) *Nature*, **257**, 149.
12. Nemazee,D.A. and Burki,K. (1989) *Nature*, **337**, 562.
13. Chace,J.H. and Scott,D.W. (1989) In *The Year in Immunology 1988.* Cruse,J.M. and Lewis,R.E. (ed.), Karger, Basle, p. 181.
14. Teale,J.M. and Klinman,N.R. (1984) *J. Immunol.*, **133**, 1811.
15. Goodnow,C.C., Crosbie,J., Adelstein,S., Lavoie,T.B., Smith-Gill,S., Brink,R.A., Pritchard-Bristoe,H., Wotherspoon,J.S., Loblay,R.H., Raphael,K., Trent,R.J., and Basten,A. (1988) *Nature*, **334**, 676.
16. Scott,D.W., Chace,J.H., Warner,G.L., O'Garra,A., Klaus,G.G.B. and Quill,H. (1987) *Immunol. Rev.*, **99**, 153.
17. Waldschmidt,T. and Vitetta,E.S. (1985) *J. Immunol.*, **134**, 1436.
18. Mitchell,G.F., Humphrey,J.H. and Williamson,A.R. (1972) *Eur. J. Immunol.*, **2**, 460.
19. Klaus,G.G.B., Abbas,A.K. and McElroy,P.J. (1977) *Eur. J. Immunol.*, **7**, 387.
20. Goodnow,C.C., Crosbie,J., Jorgensen,H., Brink,R.A. and Basten,A. (1989) *Nature*, **342**, 385.
21. McConnell,I.C.M. (1971) *Nature (New Biol.)*, **233**, 177.
22. Klaus,G.G.B. and Humphrey,J.H. (1974) *Eur. J. Immunol.*, **4**, 370.
23. Schrader,J. and Nossal,G.J.V. (1974) *J. Exp. Med.*, **139**, 1582.
24. Bretscher,P. and Cohn,M. (1970) *Science*, **169**, 1042.
25. DeFranco,A.L. (1989) *Nature*, **342**, 340.

Glossary

Accessory cell: a cell which presents antigen to T cells (and may also provide other signals necessary for T cell activation); also called antigen-presenting cells.

Adjuvant: a substance which nonspecifically enhances the immune response to an antigen.

Affinity: a thermodynamic measure of the strength of interaction between an antibody molecule and its epitope.

Affinity maturation: the increase in average antibody affinity seen with time after immunization.

Anamnestic response: heightened, more efficient response to re-immunization, produced by memory cells (q.v.).

Antigen: a substance capable of reacting with components of the immune system, such as antibody.

Avidity: the *functional* combining strength of an antibody (or receptor-bearing cell) with its antigen, which is determined by the affinity of the antibody, and its valency (or the number of receptors/cell).

CD molecules: a nomenclature (cluster determinant) describing lymphocyte differentiation antigens (cell surface markers).

Class I (II) antigens: products of the MHC (q.v.) which are involved in the presentation of peptide epitopes to T cells.

Clone: a family of cells (or organisms) which are genetically identical.

Clonal abortion: deletion of (self-reactive) clones of T or B cells during their development.

Clonal anergy: inactivation (rather than deletion) of clones of cells by antigen (tolerogen, q.v.).

Clonal selection: antigen-induced activation of clones of T and/or B cells bearing receptors for that antigen.

Cognate help: MHC-restricted (q.v.) cell contact-mediated activation of B cells mediated by T helper cells (q.v.).

65

Cytokines: soluble proteins (many produced by T cells) which act on cells of the immune system (and often other cells as well).

Epitope: a chemical configuration on an antigen which is recognized by either antibodies, or T cell receptors (also called an antigenic determinant).

Fab: single arm of an antibody, containing one combining site (cf. F(ab')$_2$.

Fc receptor: receptor binding the constant (Fc) portion of antibodies.

Germinal centre: area of B cell proliferation in follicles in secondary lymphoid organs, concerned with generation of B memory cells.

Ia antigens: murine Class II antigens (q.v.).

Idiotype: antigenic determinants associated with the variable regions of antibody (or T cell receptor) molecules.

Immunogen: an antigen which induces an immune response (cf. tolerogen, q.v.).

Interleukin: see cytokine.

Isotype: immunoglobulin class or subclass (e.g. IgM, IgG, etc.).

Isotype (or class) switching: genetically determined capacity of IgM-producing B cells to produce other isotypes, such as IgG.

Lymphokine: a cytokine (q.v.) produced by lymphocytes.

Memory cells (also called secondary cells): B or T cells which have been primed with antigen, and which produce secondary (or anamnestic, q.v.) immune responses following restimulation.

MHC (major histocompatibility complex): a gene complex encoding Class I and Class II (transplantation) antigens, which are recognized by T cells.

MHC restriction: the need for MHC compatibility during cell – cell interactions.

Plasma cell: highly differentiated antibody-secreting B cell.

Pre-B cells: precursors of B cells, which have not yet produced surface immunoglobulin receptors.

Repertoire: the total number of antibody (or T cell receptor) specificities which the immune system can make.

Self – nonself discrimination: capacity of the immune system to respond to foreign antigens, but (generally) not to components of the body.

Surface immunoglobulin: clonally distributed antigen receptors on B cells.

T cell receptor: clonally distributed antigen receptors on T cells, which are distinct from surface immunoglobulins.

T-dependent (antigen): antigens (e.g. proteins) which require the participation of T helper cells to induce responses.

T-independent (antigen): antigens such as polysaccharides, which can induce antibody responses without the aid of T cells.

T helper cells: a subpopulation of T cells which help other cells (such as B cells) to respond to antigen.

Tolerance: immunological unresponsiveness to an antigen (e.g. to self antigen).

Tolerogen: a form of an antigen which induces tolerance, rather than immunity.

Index